Emergency Medicine's Pediatric Top Clinical Problems

Dale Woolridge, MD, PhD, FACEP, FAAEM, FAAP

Introduction

This book was designed as a clinical primer on key topics in the emergent/urgent care of children. It is our hope that the emergency medicine resident or student may keep this book on their person and use it as a quick reference and quiz during a case or during down time. Each chapter is by no means a complete review and therefore offers suggestions for additional readings.

This book stemmed conceptually through combined emergency medicine/pediatrics dual training. These training programs exist within and are complimentary to categorical emergency medicine and categorical pediatric training. Combined training has, since its conception, fostered education between the two departments. It is a natural tendency for dual emergency medicine/pediatric residents to share his or her knowledge of pediatrics with their emergency medicine colleagues and to share his or her knowledge of emergency medicine with their pediatric colleagues. This book is therefore an attempt to compile the educational material and networking that is inherent to dual training.

Acknowledgements

I would like to thank my children, Anna and Garrett, who above all others keep me young and make every day exciting. I would like to thank my wife, Michelle who is forever supportive in all that I do.

I would also like to thank all those in emergency medicine, pediatrics, or both who contributed directly and indirectly to this endeavor. It has been a true pleasure to work with all of these authors. The complimentary nature of dual training in emergency medicine and pediatric has allowed me to take part in the two areas of medicine I love most. I am blessed to be able to enjoy colleagues in two departments, residents in two departments, and in the training of combined emergency medicine/pediatric residents who are also of two departments.

Dale Woolridge

Project Editor

Dale P. Woolridge, MD, PhD, FACEP, FAAEM, FAAP
Director Emergency Medicine/Pediatrics Residency Program
Associate Professor of Emergency Medicine and Pediatrics
The University of Arizona

Notice

Emergency medicine is an ever-changing field. Although every effort has been made to ensure dosages and treatment guidelines are accurate, ultimate responsibility remains with the treating physician. Neither the author nor the publisher assumes any responsibility for injury to persons or property.
Every effort has been made to follow diagnostic and therapeutic guidelines of ACEP, AHA, ACA, NIH, AHCPR, AAP, actual clinical practices, and the most recent and respected current clinical texts in pediatric medicine and emergency medicine.

Printed in the USA. ISBN: 1-929854-16-1

Additional copies of this publication are available from EMRA, 1125 Executive Circle, Irving, TX 75038-2522, 972-550-0920, www.emra.org.

Please send comments or suggestions to emra@emra.org.

EMRA Staff

Michele Byers, CAE
Executive Director

Leah Stefanini
Publications/Events Coordinator

Griffin Achilles
Administrative Assistant

Common Phone Numbers and Pagers

Admitting	______	Social Work	______
Blood Bank	______	Stress Lab	______
CCU	______	Supply	______
Chaplain	______	Urgent Care	______
Clinical Supervisor	______	Ultrasound	______
CT	______	Other	______
CT-Body	______	Other	______
CT-Neuro	______	Take-Out (Deli)	______
Case Management	______	Take-Out (Pizza)	______
Child Life	______	Take-Out ( )	______
ED Fax	______	Cardiology	______
ED UA Desk	______	CT Surgery	______
ED X-Ray	______	Dentistry/OMFS	______
EEG	______	ENT	______
EM Chief	______	Family Medicine	______
Help Desk	______	Internal Medicine	______
Information	______	Neurology	______
Lab (Chemistry)	______	Neorosurgery	______
Lab (Hematology)	______	NICU	______
Lab (Micro)	______	OB/GYN	______
Lab ( )	______	Orthopedics	______
Medical Records	______	Pediatrics (inpatient floor)	______
Nuclear Med	______	Pediatric Chief	______
OR	______	Pediatric Cardiology	______
Paging	______	Pediatric GI	______
Pathology	______	Pediatric H/O	______
Pharmacy (Inpt)	______	Pediatric ID	______
Pharmacy (Outpt)	______	Pediatric Surgery	______
Physical Therapy	______	Psychiatry	______
PICU	______	Radiology	______
Poison Control	______	Radiology Spec	______
Pulmonary Function	______	Surgery	______
Respiratory Therapy	______	Toxicology	______
Radiology Reads	______	Trauma	______
Security	______	Trauma Chief	______
SICU	______	Urology	______

Table of Contents

Acute Otitis Media

Brian D. Clothier, MD, MS
Instructor, Division of Emergency Medicine
Attending Physician, Emergency Department, Primary Children's Medical Center
University of Utah

Background

- Commonly over-diagnosed in the ED as an excuse to give antibiotics to a febrile or fussy child.
- New guidelines published in 2004 by the AAP/AAFP apply to healthy children between the ages of 2 months and 12 years.[1]
- Growing concerns over antibiotic resistance, medication side-effects, and simply practicing good medicine make it essential to get the diagnosis right the first time.

Critical Knowledge

- **Make the right diagnosis**. While purulent drainage from a perforated tympanic membrane represents obvious otitis media, the diagnosis is rarely that simple. AOM is defined by the following triad: acute onset <48 hours, middle ear effusion, and middle ear inflammation with otalgia.
  - **Acute onset <48 hours:** otitis media with effusion lasting longer than 2 days is a different diagnostic entity and does not require treatment with antihistamines, antimicrobials, corticosteroids, or decongestants.[1] Rather, a PCP should follow these chronic cases.
  - **Middle Ear Effusion (MEE):** MEE is indicated by a bulging TM, otorrhea, an air fluid level behind the TM or limited or absent TM mobility. Pneumatic otoscopy is the diagnostic modality of choice as it is the most practical for the ED physician. Clinical observance of an immobile tympanic membrane has been shown to dramatically improve the accuracy of the diagnosis of middle ear effusion.[2]
  - **Middle ear inflammation:** middle ear inflammation is indicated by erythema of the TM or otalgia and is a requirement for the diagnosis but, as stated above, is not the *sine qua non* without MEE and an onset of </= 48 hours.

Diagnostic Strategies

The entire triad must be present as described above. An immotile or poorly motile TM may be the best clue to the emergency physician that AOM exists. Taking the time to make the child feel as safe and comfortable as possible prior to otoscopy will result in a better examination. Cerumen should be cautiously removed as necessary using a 1:1 solution of peroxide and water or a curette. Take care not to introduce anything into the middle ear through a perforated tympanic membrane.

Treatment

All Children Need Pain Control

- *Acetaminophen* and topical *benzocaine* are appropriate for both infants and older children.
- *Ibuprofen* is not indicated in children less than 6 months of age because there is no evidence to support its safe use.
- Narcotic/*codeine* preparations are not recommended in the infant population because of the risk of respiratory depression and altered mental status[1] and are generally not indicated in the treatment of AOM at any age unless severe pain is present.
- Home remedies such as warm oil in the ear canal (if otorrhea is absent and the tympanic membrane is intact) or application of heat over the ear offer little or no risk and may provide additional comfort.

Some May Be Observed without Antibiotics

Meta-analysis of multiple previous studies has shown that 7 to 20 children must be treated with antibiotics for AOM in order for one to receive benefit.[4,5,6] Observation without antibiotics is an acceptable treatment for selected patients.

The AAP/AAFP Guidelines Include Recommendations Stratified by Age

- Infants less than 6 months of age should be treated with antibiotics even if the clinician is uncertain of the diagnosis.
- Children 6 months to 2 years should be treated with antimicrobials if the diagnosis of AOM is certain or if the diagnosis is uncertain but the infant's temperature is 39C or higher or there is moderate to severe otalgia.
- Well-appearing infants greater than 6 months old with an uncertain diagnosis who do not meet the requirements for fever and pain may be treated with symptomatic relief and analgesia while deferring antibiotics for 48 to 72 hours. This option mandates reliable caregivers and prompt follow-up with a PCP.

Antibiotic Choices

A variety of factors including the routine use of the heptavalent pneumococcal vaccine have changed the causative agent profile for AOM. 35% to 50% of cases of AOM are caused by nontypable H influenzae, 25% to 40% by Streptococcus pneumonae and 5% to 10% by Moraxella cateralIis. Viruses are the sole causative agent in 5 to 15% of cases, but may play a role in up to 75% of cases.[1]

- For reasons of susceptibility profile, low side effects, price and palatability, initiate antibiotic therapy with "high-dose" *amoxicillin* at 80 to 90 mg/kg/day for most children.
- *Amoxicillin-clavulanate* dosed at 90 mg/kg/day should be initiated for children with fever of 39C or higher, moderate to severe otalgia, or in cases where coverage for beta-lactamase positive Haemophilus influenza or Moraxella catarrhalis is desired.
- Children allergic to *penicillin* where the reaction is not a type I hypersensitivity reaction may be treated with a *cephalosporin* such as *cefdinir* (the most palatable), *cefuroxime*, or *cefpodoxime*. Those who do have a history of urticaria or anaphylaxis with *penicillin* may be treated with *azithromycin*, *clarithromycin*, or *trimethoprim-sulfamethoxazole*.
- *Parenteral ceftriaxone* may be given to those who cannot tolerate oral medications.[1]

Duration of Therapy

Current recommendations are for 10 days of therapy for all children under 6 years and for all seriously ill children. Older children with mild disease may be treated for 5 to 7 days.

Treatment Failures

Children who present to the ED after 48-72 hours of therapy without improvement should be thoroughly re-evaluated for other etiologies of symptoms. If the diagnosis of AOM is confirmed, their treatment should be "upgraded" by switching to high-dose *amoxicillin-clavulanate* 90 mg/kg/day or to one of the aforementioned *cephalosporins*. Those who present to the ED after failure of these treatment modalities should be treated with *parenteral cephalosporins*. Treatment with *clindamycin* should be reserved for those who fail the aforementioned regimens and for whom tympanocentesis is desired but not immediately available.[1]

Questions

1. The diagnostic triad of AOM includes all the below EXCEPT?
   A. Onset <48 hours
   B. Middle ear effusion
   C. Rhinorhea
   D. Middle ear inflammation

   Answer: C

2. What is the most common causative agent of AOM?
   A. Viruses
   B. Nontypable H influenzae
   C. Moraxella caterallis
   D. Streptococcus pneumonae

   Answer: B

3. Based on the latest AAP/AAFP recommendations, what is the treatment strategy for an otherwise healthy 18 month old with an unclear case of AOM who is only mildly ill?
   A. Oral *amoxicillin* –low dose
   B. Oral *amoxicillin* –high dose
   C. Oral *azithromycin*
   D. Observe with prompt follow-up

   Answer: D

References

1. Subcommittee on Management of Acute Otitis Media—American Academy of Pediatrics and American Academy of Family Physicians. Clinical practice guideline: diagnosis and management of acute otitis media. *Pediatrics* 2004; 113:1451-1465.
2. Jones WS, Kaleida PH. How helpful is pneumatic otoscopy in improving diagnostic accuracy? *Pediatrics* September 2003;112:510-3.
3. Rosenfeld RM, Vertrees JE, Carr J, et al. Clinical efficacy of antimicrobial drugs for acute otitis media: metaanalysis of 5400 children from thirty-three randomized trials. *Journal of Pediatrics*. 1994;124:355-367.
4. Del Mar C, Glasziou P, Hayem M. Are antibiotics indicated as initial treatment for children with acute otitis media? A meta-analysis. *British Medical Journal*. 1997; 314:1526-1529.
5. Glasziou PP, Del Mar CB, Hayem, M, Saunders SL. *Antibiotics for acute otitis media in children*. Cochrane Database Syst Rev. 2000; 4:CD000219.

Apparent Life Threatening Events (ALTE)

Sean M. Fox, MD
Emergency Medicine/Pediatrics Combined Resident
Department of Emergency Medicine and Pediatrics
University of Maryland

Critical Knowledge

- **A**pparent **L**ife **T**hreatening **E**vent (**ALTE**) is not a diagnosis, but rather a description of symptoms that generates considerable anxiety and concern for a child's caregiver.
- Definition: "An episode that is frightening to the observer and that is characterized by some combination of apnea (central or obstructive), color change (usually cyanotic or pallid, but occasionally erythematous or plethoric) marked change in muscle tone (usually marked limpness), choking, or gagging. In some cases, the observer fears that the infant has died."[1]
- ***Apnea*** is a common clinical problem in infants and can be normal or pathologic.
  - *Periodic breathing* is a normal pattern of breathing that involves three or more respiratory pauses, each being more than 3 seconds, with less than 20 seconds total duration. There is normal breathing between these episodes.
  - *Apnea of prematurity* is pathologic apnea that occurs in preterm infants and often resolves by 37 weeks gestational age.
  - *Pathologic apnea* is associated with ***cyanosis, bradycardia, abrupt marked pallor or hypotonia***, <u>or</u> being ***>20 seconds in duration.***
- Since ALTE is a collection of symptoms, the etiologies are vast and diverse.
- The evaluation in the emergency department must first look to detect any immediately life-threatening causes.
- Often the initial evaluation will be of a normal appearing child in no apparent distress, yet, a low threshold for admission is still appropriate.

Background and/or Epidemiology and/or Anatomy

- The true incidence is difficult to determine given the heterogeneity of the group that comprises it.
  - Since 1997, several studies have attempted to better describe the epidemiology of ALTE using the NIH published definition.
  - Incidence of ALTE for all infants: between 0.2% and 6%.[2,3]
  - 45% to 50% of the ALTE patients are classified as idiopathic.[4]
- Morbidity and mortality of ALTE
  - Primarily associated with the underlying etiology
  - Even idiopathic ALTE's, however, have had documented long-term neurological sequelae.[1,5] The mortality for idiopathic ALTE is classified as being between 0% and 6%.[1]
- Risk factors
  - Factors associated with an increased mortality
    - Sleep-onset of apnea requiring resuscitation
    - Similar episode prior
    - A sibling who was the victim of SIDS
    - Development of a seizure disorder during monitoring[6]
- Sudden Infant Death and Apparent Life Threatening Events
  - While similarities exist, an association between ALTE and SIDS has **<u>not</u>** been demonstrated.[1]
  - Following the initiation of the Back-to-Sleep program in 1992, there was no noted decrease in the incidence in ALTE, while the incidence of SIDS did decline.[7]

Differential Diagnosis and/or Critical Concepts

- ALTEs have a multitude of identifiable causes. Changes in color, muscle tone, and respirations may be symptoms of various specific diseases.[1,2]
  - GI (most common diagnosed pathology)
    - GERD
    - Intussusception
    - Volvulus
  - Neurologic (second most common diagnosed pathology)
    - Seizure disorder

- CNS bleed
    - Malformation/tumors
  - Respiratory (third most common diagnosed pathology)
    - Obstructive sleep apnea
    - Airway abnormalities (i.e., laryngotracheomalacia, vocal cord masses)
    - Foreign-body aspiration
  - Cardiac
    - Arrhythmias
    - Tamponade
    - Congenital heart disease
  - Metabolic
    - Dehydration and electrolyte derangements
    - Inborn errors of metabolism
    - Endocrine abnormalities
  - Infectious
    - Meningoencephalitis
    - Sepsis
    - RSV and upper respiratory infections
    - Pertussis, croup
    - Pneumonia
  - Non-accidental injuries
  - 50% of ALTE cases have no identifiable etiology[1]
- Dual diagnoses (i.e., a patient with respiratory infection and gastroesophageal reflux) may exist

Treatment/Evaluation

1. Address the ABCDE's first! Take care not to be cavalier with a patient that looks well
2. Address the most life threatening etiologies first
3. There is no advocated minimal evaluation for patients presenting as ALTE's[8]

4. The most important initial diagnostic tool is a thorough history and physical.
   - History points
     - Who was present, what was observed, and what actions were taken
     - What kind of apnea was the patient having
       - **Central apnea** - may be seen as a lack of respiratory effort
       - **Obstructive apnea** - describe choking or gagging or may even describe significant chest wall excursion efforts or abdominal wall muscle contraction without successful ventilation
       - **Mixed apnea** - signs of both central and obstructive apnea. Gastroesophageal reflux can induce bronchospasm and also alter respiratory drive by affecting chemoreceptors.
     - Previous events and their similarities and differences
     - Timing
       - Was the patient asleep?
       - Was the patient eating?
       - Was the patient playing?
     - What type of bedding was the child in and was there any co-sleeping (risk of smothering)
     - Recent illnesses and feeding difficulties
     - Recent medications given
     - Birth history, weight gain, and developmental milestones
     - History of SIDS or infants death within the family
     - Family history of cardiovascular, genetic, metabolic, or seizure disorders. Also any psychiatric illnesses should be inquired.
     - Family's social circumstances
   - Physical exam points
     - Airway, breathing, and circulation
     - A **full set of vital signs** including fingerstick as well as height and weight.

       NOTE: hypoglycemia is easily treated and can often present with symptoms that could be classified as an ALTE.
     - Dysmorphisms
     - Airway abnormalities

- Significant murmurs
- Presence of emesis
- Abdominal distension
- Hernias
- Thorough neurologic assessment including a **Fundoscopic** exam
- >50% of ALTE patients have normal initial physical examinations.[3,9,10]

5. While there is no minimal work-up, the evaluation can be rather extensive given the vast differential for ALTE.[3, 8, 11]
   - Numerous studies can prove to be beneficial when based upon the history and physical.
   - The initial assessment of ~70% of ALTE patients directed the further evaluation.[11]
     - For patients less than 1 month old, there should be a low threshold for a full sepsis work-up.
     - Patients with significant murmurs may benefit from an cchocardiogram.
     - There will be more utility in obtaining a nasopharyngeal swab for Respiratory Syncytial Virus in patients with URI signs than in those without symptoms.
     - A story that continues to change or other findings concerning for abuse would warrant a head CT to be done.
     - An abnormal fingerstick may point to an underlying genetic or metabolic pathology and should generate an appropriate work-up.
   - ~30% of ALTE patients had inconclusive histories and physicals.[11]
     - It has been found that in these patients, obtaining a white blood cell count, urinalysis and urine culture, chest x-ray, brain imaging, screening for gastroesophageal reflux, and pneumogram are the best screening tools for significant underlying pathologies.
     - In these patients, broad evaluations for systemic infections, metabolic diseases, or blood chemistry abnormalities are generally not productive.

6. Disposition
   - Most of these cases, without obvious benign etiologies, deserve a period of observation in the hospital in a monitored setting.[8, 10]
     - The presenting symptoms correlate poorly with the final diagnosis.[9]
     - It is been found that 7.8% of those who had a negative emergency department evaluation later required medical intervention while in the hospital.[10]
   - The possible extensive work-up and the emotional stress that the event and the process of evaluation places upon the family are both best relieved by admitting the patient.

Questions

1. A mother brings in her 3 week old because she found him floppy and not breathing during a nap. The patient was given rescue breaths by the mother and then returned to normal. The EMS crew reports no abnormalities. The child is alert and appears well without distress and no obvious focal findings on primary survey. What is the next most appropriate step?

   A. Head CT

   B. History and physical

   C. CBC, U/A, CXR

   D. RSV swab

   E. Admit

   Answer: B

2. A 2 week old is brought in by the parents who became concerned when she stopped breathing and turned blue. The parents note that she has not been feeding well. The infant is now alert, but jittery, tachycardic, irritable, and tachypneic. You should do which of the following first?

   A. Ask a nurse to draw a variety of blood samples and hold spare tubes

   B. Administer antibiotics

   C. Full set of vital signs including a fingerstick

   D. Bolus with 10 ml/kg of 3% *saline*

   E. Administer *prostaglandin E*

   Answer: C

References

1. *Infantile apnea and home monitoring.* National Institutes of Health Consensus Statement, 1986. 6(6): p. 1-10.
2. Brooks, J.G., *Apparent life-threatening events and apnea of infancy.* Clin Perinatol, 1992. 19(4): p. 809-38.
3. Davies, F. and R. Gupta, Apparent life threatening events in infants presenting to an emergency department. *Emerg Med J*, 2002. 19(1): p. 11-6.
4. Kiechl-Kohlendorfer, U., et al., *Epidemiology of apparent life threatening events.* Arch Dis Child, 2005. 90(3): p. 297-300.
5. Milioti, S. and C. Einspieler, *The long-term outcome of infantile apparent life-threatening event (ALTE): a follow-up study until midpuberty.* Neuropediatrics, 2005. 36(1): p. 1-5.
6. Oren, J., D. Kelly, and D.C. Shannon, *Identification of a high-risk group for sudden infant death syndrome among infants who were resuscitated for sleep apnea.* Pediatrics, 1986. 77(4): p. 495-9.
7. Gershan, W.M., N.S. Besch, and R.A. Franciosi, A comparison of apparent life-threatening events before and after the back to sleep campaign. *Wmj*, 2002. 101(1): p. 39-45.
8. Kahn, A., Recommended clinical evaluation of infants with an apparent life-threatening event. Consensus document of the European Society for the Study and Prevention of Infant Death, 2003. *Eur J Pediatr*, 2004. 163(2): p. 108-15.
9. Gray, C., F. Davies, and E. Molyneux, *Apparent life-threatening events presenting to a pediatric emergency department.* Pediatr Emerg Care, 1999. 15(3): p. 195-9.
10. De Piero, A.D., S.J. Teach, and J.M. Chamberlain, ED evaluation of infants after an apparent life-threatening event. *Am J Emerg Med*, 2004. 22(2): p. 83-6.
11. Brand, D.A., et al., *Yield of diagnostic testing in infants who have had an apparent life-threatening event.* Pediatrics, 2005. 115(4): p. 885-93.

Cardiopulmonary Resuscitation

Albert Fiorello, MD, FACEP, RDMS
Assistant Professor of Emergency Medicine
The University of Arizona

Pediatric Cardiopulmonary Arrest

Based on 2005 AHA Pediatric CPR Guidelines[1-3]

Background/Epidemiology

- Pediatric cardiopulmonary arrest is uncommon - incidence of pediatric cardiopulmonary arrest is approximately 2.6-19.7 annual cases per 100,000 pediatric population.[4]
- Most pediatric cardiopulmonary arrests are due to primary respiratory arrest or decompensated shock.
- SIDS 23%, trauma 20%, respiratory 16%, submersion 12%, cardiac 8%, CNS 6%.[5]
- Primary arrhythmia causing cardiac arrest in children is rare.
- Presenting rhythm asystole 67%, PEA 24%, ventricular fibrillation 9%.[5]
- Overall survival of pediatric out of hospital cardiac arrest is poor, about 4% overall.[4]
- Factors associated with greater overall survival include submersion injury associated arrests, witnessed arrests, and bystander CPR.[4]
- Long term survival is much greater for victims of respiratory arrest than for cardiac arrest (70% vs 21%).[6]
- The length based Broselow tape simplifies resuscitations by providing size-appropriate doses and equipment sizes.

Airway Obstruction and Management (AB of ABCs)

- In the absence of neck trauma, use a head tilt-chin lift method to open the airway.
- In the presence of possible neck trauma, use a jaw thrust method without head tilt
- If a jaw thrust method fails, attempt to use an oral or nasopharyngeal airway. If this fails and advanced airway devices are not immediately available, use the head tilt-chin lift method since maintaining an airway and providing ventilation are crucial.

- Ventilate using bag-mask ventilation. Bag-mask ventilation can usually be as effective as ventilating through an endotracheal tube for short periods and actually may be safer, especially in the pre-hospital setting.[7]
- Use a C-clamp method to provide a tight seal when using bag-mask ventilation. A two person technique is usually more effective than ventilation by a single rescuer.
- Provide high flow supplemental oxygen.
- If prolonged ventilation is necessary, consider using advanced airway techniques.
- A pediatric laryngeal mask airway may be useful for patients who are difficult to ventilate with a bag-mask or as a rescue device for failed endotracheal intubation.
- Beyond the neonatal period, both cuffed and uncuffed endotracheal tubes may be used.
- Avoid excessive ventilation. This may be detrimental because: it impedes venous return, cerebral blood flow, and coronary perfusion by increasing intrathoracic pressures; causes air trapping and barotrauma; and increases the risk of regurgitation and aspiration.
- Rapid sequence intubation is not needed in a full cardiopulmonary arrest, but may be useful in a patient with impeding respiratory arrest requiring airway management. When using RSI you must always have a backup plan for airway management in case initial attempts fail.
- After intubation, confirm ETT placement with auscultation of bilateral breath sounds and lack of gastric insufflation sounds, observation of bilateral chest wall movement, end tidal CO_2 detection, and chest x-ray.
- Initial ventilator settings: TV 10-12 ml/kg (8-10 ml/kg for asthmatics), RR age appropriate, FiO_2 100%, PEEP 3-5. Adjust settings as needed.
- After intubation, consider placement of a NG tube to decompress the stomach.
- If an intubated patient's condition suddenly deteriorates, reassess the airway **(DOPE)**
    - **D**isplacement of the tube from the trachea
    - **O**bstruction of the tube
    - **P**neumothorax
    - **E**quipment failure (if the patient was on a ventilator, take him off the ventilator and provide ventilation via bag)

Circulation and Vascular Access (C of ABCs)

Chest Compressions

- If pulses are absent, begin chest compressions.
- If despite oxygenation and ventilation, the pulse is <60 and there are signs of poor perfusion, begin chest compressions.
- "Push hard and push fast." Depress the chest approximately 1/3 to 1/2 the AP diameter of the chest at a rate of approximately 100 compressions per minute.
- Release completely after each compression to allow the chest to fully recoil.
- Minimize interruptions of chest compressions.
- For two rescuer CPR without an advanced airway in place, provide 15 compressions, followed by 2 ventilations.
- When an advanced airway is in place, provide compressions at 100 per minute and 8-10 ventilations per minute (do not pause compressions for ventilations).

Vascular Access

- Attempt placement of a peripheral IV, but limit the time of this attempt. If immediate peripheral IV access is not obtained, move on.
- Intraosseous access can be achieved rapidly and is safe and effective for administering fluids, drugs, and blood products.
- Central venous access may also be obtained, but usually takes more time than placement of an IO line.
- If attempts at vascular access fail, *naloxone, atropine, diazepam, epinephrine*, and *lidocaine* ("NAVEL") may be administered via the endotracheal tube. Optimal doses are not unknown, see table 1.
- To treat shock, give an initial bolus of 20 cc/kg of an isotonic crystalloid fluid (normal *saline* or *lactated ringers*).

Pulseless Arrest

- Presenting rhythm may be asystole, PEA, ventricular fibrillation, or ventricular tachycardia.
- Asystole and wide complex bradycardia are the most common in asphyxial arrests.

Shockable Rhythms: Ventricular Fibrillation/Pulseless Ventricular Tachycardia

- Defibrillation is the definitive treatment.
- Survival declines with increased time to defibrillation, therefore attempt defibrillation immediately.
- Perform chest compressions while preparing defibrillator.
- Use largest paddles or pads that will fit on the chest wall leaving about 3 cm between paddles (usually use adult paddles for children >10 kg or 1y, infant paddles for children <10 kg).
- If using paddles, apply electrode cream or paste. Self adhering defibrillation pads do not require additional gel.
- Place one paddle over the right side of the upper chest and the other at the apex of the heart (left of the left nipple). Apply firm pressure.
- Initial defibrillation (monophasic or biphasic) is at 2 J/kg. Subsequent attempts should be at 4 J/kg.
- Resume chest compressions immediately after delivering the shock and continue for about 5 cycles.
- Check the rhythm. If a shockable rhythm persists, give another shock at 4 J/kg and give *epinephrine* (0.01 mg/kg IV/IO = 0.1 mL/kg 1:10,000). Repeat the dose of *epinephrine* every 3-5 minutes during cardiac arrest.
- After 5 cycles of CPR, check the rhythm. If the rhythm continues to be shockable, deliver another shock at 4 J/kg, resume chest compressions, and consider administration of *amiodarone* (5 mg/kg IV) or *lidocaine* (1 mg/kg IV/IO, 2-3 mg/kg ET).
- Continue CPR for 5 cycles, check rhythm, and defibrillate if necessary.
- If at any point an organized rhythm emerges, check for a pulse and proceed accordingly.
- Throughout the resuscitation, consider treatable, reversible causes (Table 3).
- Rotate rescuers performing compressions every 2 minutes to ensure continued adequate compressions.

Nonshockable Rhythms: Asystome/PEA

- Resume chest compressions
- Administer *epinephrine* (0.01 mg/kg IV/IO = 0.1 ml/kg 1:10,000). Repeat every 3-5 minutes during cardiac arrest.
- Throughout the resuscitation, consider treatable, reversible causes (Table 3)

Bradycardia with Hemodynamic Compromise

- Treat patients with bradycardia that is causing cardiorespiratory compromise
- If the patient develops pulseless arrest, treat as described previously in the Pulseless Arrest section
- Support airway, breathing, and circulation
- Administer supplemental *oxygen*
- Attach a monitor or defibrillator
- Reassess patient to determine if cardiorespiratory compromise persists despite adequate oxygenation and ventilation. If perfusion, pulses, and respirations are normal, no emergency treatment is necessary. Proceed with further evaluation.
- If heart rate <60 beats per minute and there is evidence of poor perfusion despite adequate ventilation with oxygen, start chest compressions.
- If symptomatic bradycardia persists, administer *epinephrine* (0.01 mg/kg IV/IO = 0.1 ml/kg 1:10,000). Repeat every 3-5 minutes if needed. If bradycardia persists or if it only transiently responds to the dose of *epinephrine*, consider continuous infusion of *epinephrine*.
- If bradycardia is due to increased vagal tone, administer *atropine* (0.02 mg/kg IV/IO or 0.03 mg/kg ET).
- Consider transcutaneous pacing if bradycardia is due to heart block or sinus node dysfunction not responsive to prior treatment above, especially if it is associated with congenital or acquired heart disease.
- Throughout the resuscitation, consider treatable, reversible causes (Table 3).

Tachycardia with Hemodynamic Compromise

- If the patient develops pulseless arrest, treat as described previously in the Pulseless Arrest section.
- If pulses are palpable and the patient has signs of hemodynamic compromise, ensure airway is patent, assist ventilations if needed, administer supplemental oxygen, and attach the patient to the monitor or defibrillator.
- Assess the QRS duration. ≤0.08 seconds = narrow complex tachycardia. >0.08 seconds = wide complex tachycardia.

Narrow Complex Tachycardia (≤0.08s)

If the rhythm is sinus tachycardia, search for and treat reversible causes.

- If the rhythm is probable supraventricular tachycardia (SVT) infants usually >200, children usually >180
  - Attempt vagal stimulation unless the patient is very unstable (infants and young children: apply ice to the face; older children: carotid sinus massage or Valsalva maneuver).
  - If IV access is readily available, administer *adenosine* (0.1 mg/kg rapid IV bolus). If conversion does not occur, may repeat a double dose (0.2 mg/kg rapid IV bolus).
  - Or synchronized cardioversion may be performed at 0.5 – 1 J/kg. If conversion does not occur, this may be repeated at 2 J/kg. Sedate the patient if possible, but do not delay cardioversion in an unstable patient.
  - If conversion fails after two doses of *adenosine* or two attempts at synchronized electrical cardioversion, or SVT quickly recurs after conversion, consider the use of an antiarrhythmic prior additional attempt at conversion. *Amiodarone* or *procainamide* may be used (use extreme caution when using multiple drugs that can cause QT prolongation).

Wide Complex Tachycardia (>0.08 s)

- In the setting of hemodynamic compromise, wide complex tachycardia is usually ventricular in origin, but may be supraventricular with aberrancy.
- Treat with synchronized electrical cardioversion at 0.5 –1 J/kg. If conversion does not occur, this may be repeated at 2 J/kg.
- If conversion fails after a second shock, consider the use of an antiarrhythmic (*amiodarone* or *procainamide*) prior to a third shock.

Tachycardia with Hemodynamic Stability

- Consider consultation with an expert in pediatric arrhythmias prior to treating children who are hemodynamically stable.
- For supraventricular tachycardia, follow the algorithm above.
- For ventricular tachycardia, administer an *amiodarone* infusion slowly. If *amiodarone* is not available, *procainamide* may also be used.

Special Resuscitation Situations

Trauma

- If spinal injury is suspected, restrict the motion of the neck. Use a jaw thrust method of opening the airway if possible.
- Do not over ventilate. Over ventilation can decrease cerebral perfusion. Intentional brief hyperventilation may be used as a temporizing measure if signs of impending brain herniation develop.
- Suspect thoracic trauma in all thoracoabdominal trauma, even in the absence of obvious external injuries. Tension pneumothorax, hemothorax, and pulmonary contusions may impair breathing and cause deterioration.
- If the patient has facial trauma or has a suspected basilar skull fracture, insert an orogastric tube instead of a nasogastric tube.
- Blood pressure drops late in children. Even if the blood pressure is normal, treat signs of shock with a bolus of 20 ml/kg of normal *saline* or *lactated ringers*. Give additional 20 ml/kg boluses if signs of shock persist. After 40-60 ml/kg of crystalloid fluid, give 10-15 ml/kg of packed red blood cells. Use type specific blood if possible. If type specific blood is not available, use emergency release O-negative in females and O-negative or O-positive in males.
- Always consider intra-abdominal hemorrhage, tension pneumothorax, pericardial tamponade, and spinal cord shock in children with signs of shock. Additionally intracranial hemorrhage can cause shock in a small infant.

Toxicologic Emergencies

- *Cocaine* may cause cardiac arrhythmias. For coronary vasospasm consider *nitroglycerin*, *Benzodiazepines*, and *phentolamine*. Avoid the use of β-*blockers*, as they may potentiate marked hypertension from an unopposed α effect. For ventricular arrhythmias, consider *sodium bicarbonate* in addition to standard treatment.
- Tricyclic antidepressants may cause intraventricular conduction delays, heart block, bradycardia, prolongation of the QT interval, ventricular arrhythmias, hypotension, and seizures. Treat with *sodium bicarbonate* 1-2 mEq/kg boluses until arterial pH is >7.45 and then infuse 150 mEq $NaHCO_3$ per liter of D5W to maintain alkalosis. Do not administer *quinidine*, *procainamide*, *flecainide*, *propafenone*, *amiodarone*, or *sotalol*, as they may all exacerbate cardiac toxicity. For hypotension use normal *saline* boluses.

Epinephrine and *norepinephrine* have been shown to be more effective at raising blood pressure than *dopamine* in TCA overdose.

- *Calcium channel blockers* may cause hypotension, conduction delays, and arrhythmias. Mild hypotension may be treated with small boluses of normal *saline*. For more significant hypotension, *calcium chloride* (10%) may be administered at 20 mg/kg over 5-10 minutes, followed by an infusion of 20-50 mg/kg per hour if the initial dose was beneficial. For bradycardia and hypotension, consider a high dose vasopressor such as *norepinephrine* or *epinephrine*.
- Beta blockers may cause bradycardia, heart block, decreased cardiac contractility, hypotension, and prolonged QRS and QT intervals. High dose *epinephrine* may be effective. Consider the use of *glucagon*. Consider an infusion of *glucose* and *insulin*.
- Opiods may cause hypoventilation, apnea, bradycardia, and hypotension. Treat respiratory depression initially with assisted ventilation. *Naloxone* reverses the effects of opiods. For children less that 5 years old or less than or equal to 20 kg, administer 0.1 mg/kg IV/IO/ET. For children greater than 5 years old or over 20 kg, administer 2mg IV/IO/ET.

Questions

1. For a 20 kg child, the appropriate dose of *epinephrine* used during a cardiac arrest is

   A. 1 mg IV

   B. 0.2 mg IV

   C. 10 mg IO

   D. 0.01 mg IV

   Answer: B

2. The most common presenting rhythm in pediatric cardiac arrest is ventricular fibrillation.

   A. True

   B. False

   Answer: B

3. For 2 rescuer CPR in a patient who is not intubated, the recommended compression to ventilation ratio is
   A. 100:1
   B. 30:3
   C. 15:2
   D. 50:5

   Answer: C
4. Endotracheal intubation has been shown to be far superior to bag-mask ventilation in children for short term ventilation, especially in the pre-hospital setting.
   A. True
   B. False

   Answer: B
5. Which of the following should NOT be administered down the ET tube
   A. *Lidocaine*
   B. *Epinephrine*
   C. *Sodium bicarbonate*

   Answer: C
6. In a pediatric cardiopulmonary arrest situation, if immediate peripheral IV access cannot be obtained, a ________ line should immediately be established.
   A. Internal jugular central venous
   B. Intraosseous
   C. Femoral central venous
   D. Ultrasound guided deep brachial venous

   Answer: B
7. For treatment of ventricular fibrillation, the initial defibrillation dose is
   A. 0.5 J/kg
   B. 20 J/kg
   C. 5 J
   D. 2 J/kg

   Answer: D

8. For wide complex tachycardia with pulses, but with evidence of hemodynamic compromise, the initial synchronized cardioversion dose is
   A. 0.5-1 J/kg
   B. 10-20 J/kg
   C. 5-10 J
   D. 2-4 J/kg

   Answer: A
9. If bradycardia is suspected to be due to increased vagal tone, the following should be administered
   A. *Amiodarone*
   B. *Lidocaine*
   C. *Naloxone*
   D. *Atropine*

   Answer: D
10. A 2 year old male ingested some his grandmother's *amitriptyline*. He presents with a heart rate of 120, blood pressure of 59/42, and has a wide QRS complex on the monitor. He should be treated with
    A. *Naloxone*
    B. *Atropine*
    C. *Sodium bicarbonate*
    D. *Calcium chloride*

    Answer: C

Table 1: Helpful formulas
Uncuffed ETT size = $\frac{\text{age in years} + 4}{4}$
Cuffed ETT size = $\frac{[\,(\text{age in years}) / 4\,] + 3}{4}$
ETT placement at lip = 3 x tube size
Weight (kg) = 8 + (2 x age in years) Length based tapes such as the Broselow Tape are the most accurate at estimating weight.

Table 2: Medications for Pediatric Resuscitation and Arrythmias[2]	
Medication	**Dose**
Adenosine	0.1 mg/kg (max 6 mg) given as a rapid IV bolus Repeat: 0.2 mg/kg (max 12 mg)
Amiodarone	5 mg/kg IV/IO, repeat up to15 mg/kg (max 300 mg)
Atropine	0.02 mg/kg IV/IO 0.03 mg/kg ET*
Calcium Chloride (10%)	20 mg/kg IV/IO (2 mL/kg)
Epinephrine	0.01 mg/kg (0.1 mL/kg 1:10,000) IV/IO 0.1 mg/kg (0.1 ml/kg 1:1000) ET* (max dose 1 mg IV/IO, 10 mg ET) **Note:** no survival benefit has been demonstrated by use of high dose *epinephrine* and it actually may be harmful[8]
Glucose	0.5-1 g/kg IV/IO (D10W: 5-10 mL/kg, D25W: 2-4 mL/kg, D50W: 1-2 mL/kg)
Lidocaine	Bolus: 1 mg/kg IV/IO (max dose 100 mg) Infusion: 20-50 mcg/kg/min ET*: 2-3 mg/kg
Magnesium Sulfate	25-50 mg/kg IV/IO over 10-20 minutes, faster in torsades (max dose 2 g)
Naloxone	<5 y or ≤20 kg: 0.1 mg/kg IV/IO/ET* >5 y or >20 kg: 2 mg IV/IO/ET*
Procainamide	15 mg/kg IV/IO over 30-60 min
Sodium Bicarbonate	1 mEq/kg per dose IV/IO slowly
	*(flush with 5 ml NS, follow with 5 ventilations)

Table 3: Possible Treatable Causes of Cardiopulmonary Arrest	
Hypovolemia	**T**oxins
Hypoxia	**T**amponade (cardiac)
Hydrogen ion (acidosis)	**T**ension pneumothorax
Hypo- or Hyperkalemia	**T**hrombosis (coronary or pulmonary)
Hypoglycemia	**T**rauma
Hypothermia	

References

1. 2005 American Heart Association Guidelines for Cardiopulmonary Resuscitation and Emergency Cardiovascular Care Part 12: Pediatric Basic Life Support. *Circulation.* Dec 2005; 112 (24 Supp): IV-156 - IV-166.
2. 2005 American Heart Association Guidelines for Cardiopulmonary Resuscitation and Emergency Cardiovascular Care Part 12: Pediatric Advanced Life Support. *Circulation.* Dec 2005; 112 (24 Supp): IV-167 - IV187.
3. Highlights of the 2005 American Heart Association Guidelines for Cardiopulmonary Resuscitation and Emergency Cardiovascular Care. *Currents in Emergency Cardiovascular Care.* Winter 2005; 16 (5):1-28.
4. Donoghue AJ, Nadkarni V, Berg RA, et al. Out-of-Hospital Pediatric Cardiac Arrest: An Epidemiologic Review and Assessment of Current Knowledge. *Annals of Emergergency Medicine.* Dec 2005; 46 (6):512-522.
5. Young KD, Gausche-Hill M, McClung CD, Lewis RJ. A Prospective, Population-Based Study of the Epidemiology and Outcome of Out-of-Hospital Pediatric Cardiopulmonary Arrest. *Pediatrics.* Jul 2004; 114 (1):157-164.
6. Lopez-Herce J, Garcia C, Rodriguez-Nunez A, et al. Long-Term Outcome of Pediatric Cardiorespiratory Arrest in Spain. *Resuscitation.* Jan 2005; 64 (1):79-85.
7. Gausche M, Lewis RJ, Stratton SJ, et al. Effect of Out-of-Hospital Pediatric Endotracheal Intubation on Survival and Neurological Outcome: A Controlled Clinical Trial. *Journal of American Medical Association.* Feb 9 2000; 283(6):783-790.
8. Perondi MB, Reis AG, Paiva EF, Nadkarni VM, Berg RA. A Comparison of High-Dose and Standard-Dose *Epinephrine* in Children with Cardiac Arrest. *New England Journal of Medicine.* Apr 22 2004; 350(17):1722-1730.

Children with Special Health Care Needs

Melanie S. Heniff, MD, FACEP, FAAP, FAAEM
Assistant Clinical Professor Emergency Medicine and Pediatrics
Indiana University/Methodist Hospital
Indianapolis, IN

Developmental Disabilities/Cerebral Palsy/ Spina Bifida

Critical Knowledge

- Do not use *succinylcholine* in patients with neuromuscular disorders such as muscular dystrophy.
- Can use *succinylcholine* in patients with CP, but the effects may be prolonged.
- VP shunt malfunction can be life-threatening: consider this diagnosis in VP shunt patients who have altered mental status, headache, vomiting or coma.
- *Baclofen* pump malfunction can be life-threatening: consider the diagnosis of *baclofen* withdrawal in patients with a *baclofen* pump, altered mental status, hypotension, fever, increased spasticity, muscle rigidity and pruritis. Treat *baclofen* withdrawal with IV *Benzodiazepines* until pump can be refilled. Consider overdose of *baclofen* if patient has somnolence, respiratory depression, seizures, or coma; treat by supporting the ABCs and empty reservoir from the center of the pump.

Background

- "Special needs" = **D**evelopmental **D**isabilities (**DD**): impairments in motor function, self-care, language and cognition.
- Children with DD often have multiple associated medical problems, medications, and implanted devices (VP shunts, tracheostomies, *baclofen* pumps, and gastrostomy tubes) that must be considered.
- Many medical complications are common in patients with all types of DD.
- A consistent, organized approach with review of problems by organ system is a useful way to evaluate this complex patient population.

- Identify the patient's baseline level of function to have a basis for comparison at the time of evaluation.
- **C**erebral **P**alsy (**CP**) it the single most widespread permanent physical disability in the United States.
- **N**eural **T**ube **D**efects/spina bifida (**NTD**) are the most common major birth defects in the United States.

Management

Cerebral Palsy (CP)

- A non-progressive central motor deficit with multiple causes and manifestations
  - Musculoskeletal problems: pain, spasticity
    - Pain may be difficult to localize
    - Need to undress patient for thorough exam of skin and joints
    - At increased risk of hip subluxation due to spasticity
    - Osteopenia may result in fractures after seemingly insignificant trauma
    - Check for pressure sores
    - Increase in spasticty may come from medication withdrawal/ toxicity, *baclofen* pump malfunction, pain, UTI, constipation
  - Seizures
    - Occur in 50% of children with CP
    - Consider in altered mental status: hard to recognize seizures such as partial complex seizures or psychomotor seizures
    - Standard approach to status epilepticus
  - Pulmonary problems
    - Often due to oropharyngeal incoordination and reflux
    - Recurrent pneumonia due to aspiration, weak cough, restrictive lung disease due to scoliosis
    - Wheezing/reactive airway disease, especially in setting of aspiration, and history of prematurity
    - Tracheostomy tubes
      - Most pediatric tubes are uncuffed
      - Common complications: infection, obstruction, dislodged tube

- May temporarily replace with an **E**ndo**T**racheal **T**ube (**ETT**)*
- If replacing, have smaller tubes ready in case stoma has started to close or swelling is present
- Extend the neck and lubricate the cannula before replacing
- Assume obstruction if respiratory distress: suction, and if needed irrigate with sterile *saline*; if inner cannula may remove and clean

*Tracheostomy Tube Replacement Size Estimates	
Trach tube size	*ETT size*
Shiley 2	4-4.5
Shiley 3	4.5-5
Shiley 4	5-6
Shiley 6	7-7.5

- GI problems
  - Feeding problems (due to hypotonia, weak oropharyngeal muscles, poor swallowing ability)
  - Reflux and esophagitis common
  - Failure to thrive due to feeding problems and increased caloric needs
  - May develop rapid dehydration with mild gastroenteritis (therefore have a low threshold for labs, IV fluids, and admission)
  - Superior mesenteric artery syndrome
    - Recurrent vomiting, may be bilious
    - Due to intermittent or functional obstruction of the duodenum
    - Management: improve nutrition, prone position after meals, may need surgery
  - Gastrostomy tube problems
    - Connect to suction in a patient with vomiting or respiratory distress
    - Obstruction is most common malfunction
    - May dislodge, can develop crack, fracture, leak, and may migrate to esophagus or intestines
    - If dislodged, be careful when replacing a new g-tube (it may take 2 weeks to 3 months for a fistula to mature)

    - May use a Foley Catheter to temporarily replace g-tube, but because the catheter can migrate, it should be secured to the abdominal wall
  - Jejunostomy tubes: should be replaced by an interventional radiologist, surgeon, or gastroenterologist, but a g-tube can be temporarily inserted to keep the stoma patent
  - Excess drooling: mainly cosmetic problem, but may impair swallowing
  - Constipation
    - Often severe, chronic
    - May require hospitalization for disimpaction
    - Worsened by dehydration and meds for spasticity
    - May cause abdominal pain, rectal tears, decreased appetite, increased reflux
- GU problems
  - Hygeine problems due to lower extremity spasticity
  - Incontinence, UTIs common
- HEENT problems*:* chronic otitis media, dental caries common
- Other
  - At increased risk of child abuse
  - Mental retardation in 50-60%

Spina Bifida/Neural Tube Defects (NTD)

- Disturbance in neural plate formation during development
- Dysplastic neural elements protrude through unfused verterbral arches; may be open or closed
  - Neurologic problems
    - Arnold Chiari Malformation: prolongation of the cerebellar vermis and 4th ventricle into the c-spine
      - In over 90% patients with open NTD results in hydrocephalus requiring VP shunt
      - May develop "Chiari Crisis," vocal cord paralysis, stridor, apnea, hypoxia

- VP Shunt Malfunction
  - Young child may present with irritability, lethargy, bulging fontanelle, vomiting
  - Older child may present with HA, N/V, change in intellectual capabilities, cardiovascular instability, seizures, apnea, coma
  - 1st evaluate for "routine" etiologies of symptoms (i.e., more likely causes of symptoms such as viral syndrome, otitis media, febrile illness), but consider shunt malfunction in differential
  - CT scan most useful for diagnosing if there is a prior study for comparison
  - Shunt tap most definitive test
  - Infection most common in 1-2 months after placement
  - Seizures occur in 14-29% NTD patients

- Musculoskeletal problems
  - Lower extremity weakness or paralysis
  - Bowel or bladder dysfunction
  - At risk of hip subluxation
  - Increased risk of pathologic fracture, often with increased systemic response to pain (fever, tachycardia, hypertension, or hypotension)
  - Foot deformities
  - Scoliosis
- GU problems

  Over 90% NTD patients have significant urologic problems (incontinence, UTI)
- GI problems

  Constipation is common
- Other
  - Dental caries
  - Skin breakdown
  - May be difficult intubation due to short trachea
  - Latex allergy extremely common

Questions

1. Symptoms of VP shunt malfunction can include which of the following?
   A. Headache
   B. Vomiting
   C. Altered mental status
   D. A and C
   E. All of the above

   Answer: E
2. Medical problems that children with spina bifida are predisposed to include all of the following EXCEPT?
   A. UTI
   B. Hip subluxation
   C. Seizures
   D. Bowel obstruction
   E. Latex allergy

   Answer: D

References

1. Teoh, DL. Tricks of the trade: assessment of high-tech gear in special needs children. *Clin Ped Emerg Med* 3:62-75, 2002.
2. Caterino, JM, Scheatzle, MD, and D"Antonio, JA. Descriptive analysis of 258 emergency department visits by spina bifida patients. *J Emerg Med* 31(1):17-22, 2006.
3. Green, L, Greenberg, GM, and Hurwitz, E. Primary care of children with cerebral palsy. *Clinics in Fam Pract* 5(2), 2003.
4. Abbott, R. Neurosurgical management of abnormal muscle tone in childhood. *Ped Clinics N Amer* 51(2), 2004.
5. Clark, SL and Hankins, GD. Temporal and demographic trends in cerebral palsy-fact and fiction. *Amer J Obst Gyn* 188(3), 2003.
6. Zuckerbraun, NS, Ferson, S, Albright, A, et al. Intrathecal baclofen withdrawal: emergent recognition and management. *Ped Emerg Care* 20(11), 2004.
7. Kuban, K and Leviton, A. Cerebral palsy. *N Engl J Med* 330:188-196, 1994.
8. Heniff, M. Emergency department management of children with cerebral palsy. *Ped Emerg Med Reports* 3(4), 1998.

Closed Head Injury

Mary Thiessen, MD
Attending Emergency Medicine
St. Luke's Hospital of Kansas City
Kansas City, MO

Critical Knowledge/Action

- ABCD's FIRST, immobilize C-spine
- Primary aim is to prevent secondary brain damage (hypoxia, hypoperfusion, hypercarbia)
- Establish baseline neurological function and evaluate any change in mental status
- Physical findings suggestive of intracranial injury (ICI) include: location and size of scalp hematoma, signs of basilar skull fracture, fontanel fullness, pupil size, peds GCS
- Abnormal neurologic function suggestive of **T**raumatic **B**rain **I**njury (**TBI**) include: headache, vomiting, drowsiness, irritability, amnesia, visual disturbance, focal neurologic signs, altered consciousness, signs of fractured skull
- For severe trauma requiring RSI, consider pretreatment with *atropine* 0.02 mg/kg IV and *lidocaine* 1 mg/kg IV

Epidemiology/Physiology

- Common mechanisms: falls, MVA, lack of helmet, inflicted head injury
- Impact, acceleration-deceleration, and rotational forces may cause skull and scalp injuries, neural tissue damage, or cerebral vasculature injuries.[1]
- Parietal bone is the most commonly fractured skull bone, followed by occipital, frontal and temporal bones.
- Younger age can be a strong criterion for identifying risk of ICI, especially children less than 2 years-old. [2]

Concussion/Grading/Re-injury Syndrome

- As defined by the **A**merican **A**cademy of **N**eurology (**AAN**), a concussion is "a trauma-induced alteration in mental status that may or may not involve loss of consciousness." Confusion and amnesia are hallmarks of concussion. [3]

- "Second imp act syndrome" refers to when an athlete sustains a second head injury before symptoms associated with the first injury have fully cleared. Many reports of complications (increased ICP and brainstem herniation) and even death have been attributed to second impact syndrome. However, the diagnosis remains controversial. To prevent second impact syndrome, popular guidelines recommend that athletes not return to play until the postconcussive symptoms have resolved.[3,4,5,6]
- Postconcussive symptoms refers to constellation of acute symptoms after minor head injury: somatic (headache, dizziness, blurriness), emotional (anxiety, irritability), and cognitive (concentration and memory)[7]
- How many concussions are too many? A history of multiple concussions has been associated with reduced cognitive performance on neuropsychologic testing of athletes. Deficits in executive functioning and speed of information processing have been observed.

Concussion Grading Schemes

Cantu	American Academy of Neurology	Colorado Medical Society
Grade 1 (mild)	*Grade 1*	*Grade 1*
– No LOC – PTA ≤30min	– No LOC – Transient confusion – Symptoms resolve ≤15 min	– No LOC – Transient confusion – No PTA
Grade 2 (moderate)	*Grade 2*	*Grade 2*
– LOC ≤5 min, or – PTA ≥30 min	– No LOC – Transient confusion – Symptoms last ≥15 min	– No LOC – Confusion with PTA
Grade 3 (severe)	*Grade 3*	*Grade 3*
– LOC ≥5 min, or – PTA ≥24 hrs	– Any LOC, brief or prolonged	– LOC of any duration

Scales differ on presence or length of LOC, post-traumatic amnesia (PTA), and confusion.[4,5,10]

Non-accidental Head Injuries

- Approximately 80% of deaths caused by TBI in children younger than 2 years can be attributed to inflicted head injury.[8]
- Victims of inflicted TBI tend to: be younger in age, with the majority in their first year of life, have a history of prematurity and preinjury medical problems, no mechanism offered by the caregiver, worse outcomes, more severe injuries and higher mortality rate, and boys are more commonly affected than girls.
- Children with missed inflicted head injury are younger and more commonly mis-diagnosed with accidental head injury or viral gastroenteritis. In one study, 25% of those children in the missed head injury group were re-injured before being appropriately diagnosed, and 9% of the children with missed inflicted head injury died.[9]

Differential Diagnosis/Critical Concepts

Pediatric GCS

Eye Opening	Verbal	Motor
4 - Spontaneous	**5** - Smiles/coos or appropriate words; oriented	**6** - Spontaneous movement
3 - To verbal stimuli	**4** - Irritable cries, but consolable; confused	**5** - Withdraws to touch
2 - To pain	**3** - Persistent cries to pain and not consolable	**4** - Withdraws to pain
1 - No response	**2** - Moans or grunts to pain	**3** - Abnormal flexion to pain
	1 - No response	**2** - Abnormal extension
		1 - No response

Neuroimaging

- CT scan is the imaging study of choice. If CT is not available, then skull radiographs can provide screening information, especially for infants with scalp hematomas who are at greater risk of skull fracture.[10]
- Neuroimaging studies have found subdural hemorrhage and subarachnoid hemorrhage more frequently in children with inflicted TBI; whereas epidural hemorrhage occurs more frequently in noninflicted TBI.[11,12]

Treatment

- Airway protection with orotracheal intubation
- C-spine immobilization
- Appropriate neurosurgical involvement from the beginning of treatment
- IVF resuscitation with NS or LR
- Mild hyperventilation ($PaCO_2$ ~35)
- Elevated HOB 20-30° to optimize venous drainage
- *Mannitol* 0.5-1 g/kg IV to lower ICP (may worsen hypovolemia)
- ICP monitoring
- Seizure prophylaxis: 2004 RCT studied *phenytoin* vs placebo in 102 patients 16 years old or less with moderate to severe head injuries. The study did not find a significant difference in the rate of early posttraumatic seizure in the *phenytoin* vs placebo group. [13]
- Continuous reassessment of all parameters
- Disposition: children with normal CT imaging and normal neurologic assessments after minor head trauma are at low risk for subsequent intracranial bleeding or neurologic sequelae. This low-risk subset of head-injured children may be discharged from ED if a competent caregiver is available and able to return to the ED if there is any neurologic change. Moderate to high-risk head-injured children should be admitted to trauma/neurosurgery.

Complications/Rehab

- Studies on short-term outcome show symptoms (dizziness, mood swings, temper outbursts, aggressive behavior) are more significantly reported across the injury severity spectrum.
- Children with continued problems past several months tend to have history of previous head injury, neurologic or psychiatric problems, learning or behavior difficulties, or family stressors. These "at risk" children with potential for poorer outcome should be identified and monitored for follow-up and provided resources and coping strategies. [14]
- Studies on long-term outcome are more controversial. Comprehensive review concluded that children with minor head injury may have mild but transitory alteration in cognitive functioning (attention and memory) but no reliable changes in academic or psychologic functioning. [15]

Questions

1. Which of the following is not a physical sign of underlying basilar skull fracture?
   A. CSF rhinorrhea/otorrhea
   B. Ecchymosis over the mastoid bone (Battle's Sign)
   C. Large, boggy occipital hematoma
   D. Hemotympany
   E. Periorbital ecchymosis (raccoon eyes)

   Answer: C
2. What are the potential complications associated with a basilar skull fracture?
   A. Permanent hearing loss
   B. CSF fistulas
   C. Recurrent pharyngitis
   D. Physical growth delay
   E. A and B

   Answer: E
3. All of the following tests should be ordered to rule out non-accidental head injury EXCEPT?
   A. CT and/or MRI
   B. Skeletal survey
   C. Ophthalmologic evaluation
   D. Skull radiographs
   E. Coagulation studies

   Answer: D

References

1. Savitsky, EA, Votey, SR. Current controversies in the management of minor pediatric head injuries. *Am J Emerg Med* 2000;18 (1):96-101.
2. Gruskin KD, Schutzman SA. Head trauma in children younger than 2 years: are there predictors for complications? *Arch Pediatr Adolesc Med* 1999;153:15-20.
3. Quality Standards Subcommittee, American Academy of Neurology. Practice parameter: the management of concussion in sports (summary statement). *Neurology* 1997;48 (3):581-5.

4. Kelly JP, Nichols JS, Filley CM, et al. Concussion in sports: guidelines for the prevention of catastrophic outcome. *JAMA* 1991;266 (20):2867-9.
5. Colorado Medical Society. *Report of the sports medicine committee: guidelines for the management of concussions in sport* (revised). Denver: Colorado Medical Society; 1991.
6. Cantu RC. Second impact syndrome. *Clin Sports Med* 1998;17 (1):37-44.
7. Thompson MD, Irby Jr JW. *Recovery from mild head injury in pediatric populations.* Semin Pediatr Neurol 2003;10 (2):130-9.
8. Bruce DA, Zimmerman RA. Shaken impact syndrome. *Pediatr Ann* 1989;18:482-94.
9. Jenny C, Hymel KP, Ritzen A, et al. Analysis of missed cases of abusive head trauma. *JAMA* 1999;282 (7):621-6.
10. Quayle KS, Jaffe DM, Kupperman N, et al. Diagnostic testing for acute head injury in children: when are head computed tomography and skull radiographs indicated? *Pediatrics* 1998;99 (5):1-8.
11. Ewing-Cobbs L, Kramer L, Prasad M, et al. Neuroimaging, physical, and developmental findings after inflicted and noninflicted traumatic brain injury in young children. *Pediatrics* 1998;102:300-7.
12. Keenan HT, Runyan DK, Marshall SW, et al. A population-based comparison of clinical and outcome characteristics of young children with serious inflicted and noninflicted traumatic brain injury. *Pediatrics* 2004;114:633-9.
13. Young KD, Okada PJ, Sokolove PE, et al. A randomized double-blinded placebo-controlled trial of *phenytoin* for the prvention of early posttraumatic seizures in children with moderate to severe blunt head injury. *Ann Emerg Med* 2004;43 (4):435-46.
14. Ponsford J, Willmott C, Rothwell A, et al. Impact of early intervention on outcome after mild traumatic brain injury in children. *Pediatrics* 2001;108 (6):1297-303.
15. Satz P, Zaucha K, Light R, et al. Mild head injury in children and adolescents: a review of studies (1970-1995). *Psychol Bull* 1997;122 (2):107-31.

Congenital Heart Defects

Dale P. Woolridge, MD, PhD, FACEP, FAAEM, FAAP
Director Emergency Medicine/Pediatrics Residency Program
Associate Professor of Emergency Medicine and Pediatrics
The University of Arizona

Critical Concepts

- It is not critical to determine the exact cardiac defect at hand in the emergency setting. It **is** critical, although to determine the hemodynamics at hand to be able to administer appropriate care.
- Left→right shunt lesions manifest in infancy with CHF (large cardiac lesions), or in adolescents or later with symptoms of pulmonary hypertension (small cardiac lesions).
- The hemodynamic effects of left→right shunt lesions are blunted by the high pulmonary vascular resistance in the newborn. Symptoms become more evident after one month of life when this resistance drops.
- Transient cyanosis associated with crying may suggest pulmonary disease or a cardiac defect allowing right-to-left shunting. Very often one will see the patient with a cyanotic heart defect to be "comfortably blue" at rest only to worsen with agitation. On the other hand, patients with primary pulmonary processes will show cyanosis that improved with crying since the underlying defect is ventilatory in nature.
- *Prostaglandin* therapy can have complicating side effects but should not be avoided since this therapy is lifesaving for the newborn in shock from a ductal dependent lesion.

Background

Cardiac malformation accounts for approximately 10% of infant mortality and almost all deaths.[1] The presentation of **C**ongenital **H**eart **D**isease (**CHD**) can be quite deceiving for two very important reasons. First, the diagnosis is relatively uncommon with an approximate incidence of 4 to 6 cases in 1,000 livebirths.[2] Second, neonates with congential heart disease are not always overtly symptomatic at birth and the diagnosis may be overlooked in the nursery.[3]

The age when symptoms develop can serve as a valuable tool in discerning the underlying cardiac defect at hand. Patients who develop symptoms in the first week of life tend to have ductal dependent lesions. The next crucial time at which these patients present is marked by the fall in **P**ulmonary **V**ascular **R**esistance (**PVR**) and progressive left-to-right shunting (2-6 weeks of life). Patients that present at this time are those who have lesions that allow shunting in the face of unrestricted pulmonary blood flow. Examples that are typical of this scenario include transposition of the great arteries, total anomalous pulmonary venous return and truncus arteriosus. In each of these, PVR decreases and left-to-right shunting increases which results in progressively increased pulmonary perfusion. This results in pulmonary congestion and signs of congestive heart failure. To confound matters the patient with a left-to-right shunt lesion is more susceptible to respiratory infections. Often it is an underlying infection that tips the patient into the decompensated state that requires medical care in the emergency setting.

It is not critical to determine the exact cardiac defect at hand in the emergency setting. This will be determined later after echocardiographic imaging and cardiac catheterization is performed. It is, although, critical to determine the hemodynamics at hand to be able to administer appropriate care. One of the better categorization schemes for congenital cardiac lesion is to organize by the hemodynamic manifestation of these lesions. This, physiologic categorization scheme is based on the presence or absence of hypoxia and the presence or absence of pulmonary overperfusion.

Table 1: Physiologic Classification of Congenital Heart Disease
Acyanotic Left → Right Shunt Lesions   Left Outflow Tract Obstruction ▸ Coarctation of the Aorta ▸ Aortic Stennosis ▸ Hypoplastic Left Heart ▸ Interupted Aortic Arch
Cyanotic Decreased Pulmonary Blood Flow (Right → Left Shunt Lesions) ▸ Tetralogy of Fallot ▸ Pulmonary Stenosis ▸ Pulmonary Atresia with VSD ▸ Pulmonary Atresia without VSD (Hypoplastic Right Heart) ▸ Tricuspid Atresia
Increased Pulomnary Blood Flow (Abnormal Intracardiac Mixing) ▸ **T**ranspotition of the **G**reat **A**rteries (**TGA**) ▸ **T**runcus **A**rteriosus (**TA**) ▸ **T**otal **A**nomalous **P**ulmonary **V**enous **R**eturn (**TAPVR**)

Assessment

- History
- Note genetic syndromes associated with congenital heart disease (Table 2)
- Fussiness
- Inadequate weight gain
- Low-grade fever (owed to their hyper-metabolic state)
- Feeding intolerance (feeding for the infant is equivalent to exercise in adults)
  - Length of feedings
  - Sweating during feeds
  - Taking frequent breaks

Physical Findings

- General appearance
- Varies from consolable, irritable to lethargy
- Dehydration and/or muscle wasting may be present
- Cyanosis: distinguish between cyanosis of central (always pathologic) and peripheral (may be a normal finding) (Table 3).
- Vital signs
- Respiratory rate (an increased work of breathing, although sometimes subtle, is almost always present)
- Increased heart rate
- Hypotension (late and ominous finding)
- Pre-cordial exam
- Presence and location of a precordial thrill or impulse
- Nature of S1 and S2 heart sounds
- Characteristic and timing of audible murmurs
  - Concerning findings: harshness, louder than a grade 3, thrill, hyperdynamic precordium
  - Diastolic murmurs are always abnormal
- Abdomen exam
- In CHD, hepatomegaly is much more likely to be seen in an infant than jugular venous distention and isolated lower extremity edema
- Extremities

- Varying extremity pulses (i.e., decreased lower extremity pulses in coarctation of the aorta)
- Blood pressures should be measured in the right arm (pre-aortic arch) and lower extremity (post-aortic arch)

Table 2: Genetic Syndromes with Known Association to Congenital Heart Disease	
Trisomy 21	Endocardial cushion defects
Turner's (XO)	Coarctation of the aorta
Noonan's	Pulmonary stenosis
DiGeorge	Conotruncal abnormalities (truncus arteriosus, Tetralogy of Fallot, interrupted aortic arch)
Williams	Supra-valvular insufficiency, mitral valve prolapse
Holt-Oram	Atrial septal defects

Table 3: Central vs Peripheral Cyanosis
• Peripheral cyanosis: manifestation of inadequate peripheral perfusion ▸ Blue discoloration of the hands, feet, and circumoral region ▸ Common in the neonate and generally is not indicative of a serious illness
• Central cyanosis is always abnormal ▸ May be secondary to a cardiac, pulmonary, or central nervous system etiology ▸ Blue discoloration of the trunk, extremities, lips, and mucosal membranes

Evaluation/Tests

- Pulse oximetry: pre- (right arm) and post- (either leg) ductal oxygen saturation
- Blood gas
    - Acidosis suggests inadequate oxygenation in cyanotic lesions or inadequate perfusion in acyanotic lesions
    - pCO2
        - Patients with CHD in the absence of respiratory failure are unlikely to be hypercarbic (pCO2 >40 mm Hg)

        - Most often these patients will have increased ventilation at baseline demonstrated by a pCO_2 of 25-40 mm Hg
- 100% oxygen test: administering 100% *oxygen* and assessing the rise in arterial oxygenation
    - Theory: hypoxia secondary to pulmonary disease or hypoventilation is more likely to be overcome with 100% *oxygen* while cyanotic cardiac defects that have a mixing of saturated and desaturated blood are less likely to be overcome with 100% *oxygen*
        - pO_2 value <100 mm Hg on 100% inhaled *oxygen* is highly suggestive that the cause of cyanosis IS cardiac in nature
        - pO_2 value >150 mm Hg on 100% inhaled *oxygen* is highly suggestive that the cause of cyanosis is NOT cardiac
        - pO_2 value >100 mm Hg but <150 mm Hg despite 100% *oxygen* is equivocal
- Chest radiograph
- Evaluate
    - Size and shape of the cardiac silhouette
    - Almost all congenital heart defects excluding total anomalous pulmonary venous return will result in cardiomegaly
    - "Boot shaped" in Tetralogy of Fallot
    - "Egg on a string" in transposition of the great arteries
    - "Figure 8" in total anomalous pulmonary venous return
    - Right-sided aortic arch seen in Tetralogy of Fallot and transposition of the great arteries
        - In a normal radiograph the airway will deviate slightly to the right above the carina
        - In a right-sided aortic arch the airway will be either straight or deviate to the left
    - Increased pulmonary vascular markings suggest pulmonary over-perfusion
    - Decreased pulmonary vascular markings suggest right heart obstructive lesions
- Electrocardiogram
    - Infants are born with a rightward axis (~90-180°) that converts by approximately 3-4 weeks of life to the axis more often seen in adults (~0-90°)

- Upright T-wave in V1 is normal at birth but should not persistence beyond three days of age
- Chamber hypertrophy (reference tables: criteria for hypertrophy varies by age)
- See Table 4 for a summary of concerning EKG changes

- Echocardiogram and cardiac catheterization are required for diagnosis and characterization of the altered hemodynamics

Table 4

Right Atrial Enlargement

- Peaked P waves >3 mm in any lead

Left Atrial Enlargement

- P wave duration >0.10 sec OR
- P wave with notching or plateau contour OR
- Terminal or deeply inverted P wave in V3R or V1

Right Ventricular Hypertrophy

- R wave amplitude in V1 >98%** OR
- S wave amplitude in V6 >98%** OR
- Upright T wave in V1 after 3 days of age

Right Ventricular Hypertrophy in the Newborn

- Pure R wave in V1 >10 mm OR
- R in V1 >25 mm or R in a VR >8 mm OR
- Right axis deviation >180 degrees OR
- Any Q wave in V1

Left Ventricular Hypertrophy

- R wave amplitude in V5 or V6 >98%** OR
- S wave amplitude in V1 >98%** OR
- R wave in V1 or V2 <5% OR
- Inverted T wave in V6 OR
- Q wave >4 mm in V5 or V6

Due to physiologic axis changes that naturally occur in utero, the above criteria are not as reliable in the premature infant. Criteria may not be applicable in the event of incorrect lead placement, abnormal conduction, abnormal cardiac positions, or complex cardiac detects.

**Amplitudes vary with the age of the patient and are derived from population based studies and can be obtained from published tables.

Management

- Immediate pediatric cardiology consult when congenital heart disease is expected
- "ABC's"
- Consider antibiotics: sepsis is a much more common cause of shock!
- Infants who present in the first week of life are almost exclusively ductal dependent lesions
- Treatment strategy is to maintain ductal patency
- Intravenous PGE1 (ductal dependent lesions)
    - Continuous infusion at 0.05 to 0.2 mcg/kg/min. Initiated at 0.1 mcg/kg/min
    - Consultation with a pediatric cardiologist is advisable
    - Intravenous prostaglandins are life saving in the presence of a ductal dependent lesion
    - The physician who strongly suspects the presence of an underlying ductal dependent defect in this age group should not hesitate to start prostaglandins
    - Side effects: hyperpyrexia (14%), apnea (9%-12%), and flushing (10%), tachycardia, bradycardia, hypotension
        - Close monitoring is essential
        - Strong consideration should be given to intubation prior to transfer
- Hypotension
    - Crystaloid volume bolus (10-20 ml/kg)
    - Positive inotropic agents such as *dobutamine* and/or *dopamine* (not as effective in an acidosis)
- Correcting hypoglycemia (10 cc/kg of 10% *glucose* solution)
- Correct acidosis: ventilation, fluid resuscitation, *sodium bicarbonate* (0.5-1 mEq/kg)
- Positive pressure ventilation will help with pulmonary edema but may antagonize issues of hypotension
- Consultation with a pediatric cardiologist and intensivist
- Definitive diagnosis will require echocardiography and/or cardiac catheterization

Specific Treatment

Congestive Heart Failure

- Treatment directed at decreasing afterload and increasing cardiac output
- *Furosemide* (0.5-1 mg/kg IV)
- Ace Inhibitor (consider *enalapril* 0.005-0.01 mg/kg IV)
- Inotropic agents (consider *dobutamine* ggt)

Hypoplastic Left Heart Syndrome

- *Prostaglandins IV*
- Therapy is directed at increasing pulmonary vascular resistance to promote right→left shunting across the PDA in order to promote systemic perfusion.
  - An increased PVR is promoted through hypercarbia and hypoxia
  - Ventilate to target respiratory acidosis: pCO_2 ~35
  - Oxygen restriction (target SaO_2 <90%) may require N_2 mixing into ventilator system

Hyper Cyanotic "TET" Spell

- **Theory**: muscular component of pulmonary stenosis is dynamic resulting in acute increases in obstruction to flow. Decreases in SVR (dehydration, vagal tone, etc.)
- Treatment is directed at increasing SVR and promoting flow to the lungs
  - Squatting/babies knees to chest
  - IVF boluses
  - *Morphine* (thought to decrease pulmonary obstruction)
  - *Phenylephrine* 0.1 mg/kg/dose IV/IM

Post-operative Patients

- The key to therapy is to understand the hemodynamic physiology at hand.
  - This requires a general understanding of the patient's anatomy and surgical repair process. (Common surgical repair procedures are listed in Table 5.)
  - Rely heavily on the patient's guardian who often times is very knowledgeable about their child.
- All post-operative patients are at risk for dysrhythmia. This is especially true for Tetralogy of Fallot where surgical repair requires instrumentation of the ventricle.

- Dysrhythmia is highest in the early post-operative period but can occur years later.
- Determine when medications were last adjusted. Growing children will outgrow their doses. (i.e., patients with left→right shunt lesions taking diuretics)

Table 5	
Procedure	**Description**
Blalock-Taussig	Shunt anastomosis of subclavian to pulmonary artery.
Fontan	Total cavo-pulmonary shunt. Results in redirecting systemic venous return directly to the pulmonary artery. Final stage in surgery for single ventricles.
Mustard	Atrial switch using prosthetic material for intra-atrial baffle.
Senning	Atrial switch using native material for intra-atrial baffle.
Norwood	Palliative procedure in HLHS. Involves reconstruction of hypoplastic aorta.
Ross	Transplantation of pulmonary valve to correct defective aortic HLHS valve followed by conduit from right ventricle to pulmonary artery.
Atrial septostomy	Catheter-mediated balloon dilation of foramen ovale with resultant disruption of atrial septum.
Bi-directional Glenn or Hemi-fontan	Anastomosis of superior vena cava to right pulmonary artery.
Arterial switch	Correction of TGA where aortic trunk is reconnected to the LV and the pulmonic trunk is reconnected to the RV.
Rastelli	Patch closure of VSD with conduit connecting right ventricle to pulmonary artery.

Questions

1. A hypercyanotic "Tet" spell is treated with all the following EXCEPT?

   A. *Morphine*

   B. *Phenylephrine*

   C. *Ace Inhibitors*

   D. Squating

   Answer: C

2. All of the following are true for Ventricular Septal Defects EXCEPT?
   A. Left→right shunt lesions
   B. Present acutely in the newborn period with cyanosis
   C. May cause recurrent lower respiratory infections
   D. Can present in adolescents with pulmonary hypertension.
   Answer: B

References

1. Abu-Harb, Death in infancy form unrecognized CHD, *Arch Dis Child* 1994.
2. Ferencz C, CHD prevalence at livebirth, *Am J of Epi* 121(1) 1985.31-36 & Grabitz R CHD incidence in the 1st year of life *Am J Epid* 128(2) 1988.381-388 & Richmond, Early diagnosis of congenital heart disease, Semin Neon 2001 & Ainsworth: *Arch Dis child*, Jan 1999 & Wren ADC Presentation of CHD in infancy, ADC 99 vol 80 & Kidd S The incidence of CHD in the 1st year *J of Pae* 29(5). 1993
3. Abu Harb, Presentation of obstructive L heart, *Arch Dis Child* 1994 & Ainsworth: *Arch Dis child*, Jan 1999 & Richmond, Early diagnosis of congenital heart disease, Semin Neon 2001
4. Link KM, Loehr SP, Martin EM. et al. *Congenital heart disease*. Coron Artery Dis. 1993; 4: 340-344.
5. Lin AE: Congenital heart defects in malformation syndromes. *Clin Perinatol* 1990;17:641-673.
6. Pelech AN. Evaluation of the pediatric patient with a cardiac murmur. *Pediatr Clin N Am* 1999; 46:167-188.
7. Moss AJ, Clues in diagnosing congenital heart disease. *West J Med.* 1992;156:392-398.
8. Horton LA, Mosee S, Brenner J. Use of the electrocardiogram in a pediatric emergency department. *Arch Pediatr Adolesc Med.* 1994;148:184-188.
9. Flynn PA, Engle MA, Ehlers KH, Cardiac issues in the pediatric emergency department. *Pediatr Clin N Am* 1992; 39:955-968.
10. Baïrone, MA. (ed): *The Harriet Lane Handbook.*, 14th ed., Mosby, Baltimore, MD, 1996, p. 137-138.
11. Driscoll DJ, Left to right shunt lesions. *Pediatr Clin N Am* 1999; 46:355-368.
12. Pelech AN: The cardiac murmur. *Pediatr Clin N Am.* 1998; 45:107-122.

Pathologic Condition: Gastroenteritis

Lisa Doyle, MD
Attending Physician
Utah Emergency Physicians

Critical Knowledge

- The term gastroenteritis only applies to children with nausea, vomiting AND diarrhea. Do not diagnose a child who has only nausea and vomiting with gastroenteritis. Look further for a cause of their illness.
- Dehydration is the main concern.
- Gastroenteritis is a diagnosis of exclusion in infants under 3 months of age.

Background and/or Epidemiology

- In the USA and most of the developed world, gastroenteritis is caused by self-limited viral infections (Norwalk virus, Rotavirus, enteric Adenovirus).
- Most etiologic agents that cause gastroenteritis are highly contagious via fecal-oral transmission. The major exception is Staphylococcal food poisoning.
- Contaminated food (Shigella, Staphylococcus, Norwalk virus, Vibrio species), contaminated water (Giardia, Shigella, Norwalk virus, Vibrio species), and undercooked meat (Campylobacter jejuni, E.coli, Salmonella) are other sources of exposure.
- Regardless of the infectious agent, acute gastroenteritis causes inflammatory changes to the bowel mucosa which decrease the absorptive capacity of the GI tract. This leads to significant fluid loss in the stool. Fasting due to nausea and vomiting worsens the ability of the inflamed bowel to absorb fluid.

Differential Diagnosis

- Viral gastroenteritis is a clinical diagnosis. Hallmarks are nausea, vomiting, watery diarrhea, and fever.
- Severe abdominal pain is not typically seen in acute gastroenteritis. Be sure to evaluate for an acute surgical cause of the patient's symptoms (i.e., appendicitis).
- The most common causes of bloody stool (either gross or occult) are Shigella and E.coli 0157:H7. This is the variant associated with hemolytic uremic syndrome.

- Check immediately for hypoglycemia in a child with altered mental status.

Treatment

- Rehydration. The goal is to replace the fluid loss over 4 hours.

Estimation of Dehydration Severity

Mild (3-5%)	Moderate (6-9%)	Severe (>10%)
Well-appearing, normal vital signs (slighty increased heart rate), normal to slightly decreased urine output	Ill-appearing, tachycardic, tachypneic, normal blood pressure, capillary refill <4 seconds, cool skin, sunken eyes, prolonged skin turgor, decreased tears, tacky mucous membranes, decreased urine output	Toxic appearing, tachycardic, tachypneic, hypotensive, decreased pulses, capillary refill >4 seconds, mottled skin, absent tears, dry mucous membranes, minimal urine output

% Dehydration = (Pre-illness weight – current weight/ Pre-illness weight) x 100

- Use oral rehydration in cases of mild to moderate dehydration. Use intravenous fluids in cases of severe dehydration or oral failure.
- Start with 5 ml-30ml every 5-15 minutes for the first hour. The goal is to replace 10 ml/kg in this first hour. Then, increase the intake as tolerated to reach the goal of replacing the fluid deficit in the first 4 hours.

Oral Rehydration Solution (ORS) Options

World Health Organization ORS	Recommended for all ages
Commercial ORS (Pedialyte)	Recommended or all ages
Sports drink (Gatorade)	Not recommended for kids <2years
Soda	Not recommended
Water	Not recommended
Juice*	Not recommended due to high osmotic load from *glucose*

*Dilution with ½ water and ½ juice yields a more acceptable *glucose* concentration

- Antiemetics may be used as an adjunct to oral rehydration. Ondansetron (0.15 mg/kg PO/IV; max 4 mg) has been studied with good results.
- Rehydrate with normal *saline* or *lactated ringers* at a rate of up to 40 ml/kg in the first 1-2 hours. Then convert to oral rehydration or an IV solution containing dextrose.

Intravenous Rehydration Rules

- Hemodynamically unstable patients should receive one or more 20 ml/kg boluses of isotonic crystalloid or colloid irrespective of the type of dehydration.
- IV fluids must be tailored to any electrolyte abnormalities that may be present.
- Daily requirements: Na^+ (3-4 mEq/kg/day); K^+ (1-2 mEq/kg/day)
- Maintenance fluids = daily requirement + deficit + ongoing losses.
- Use the 4:2:1 rule to calculate hourly maintainance.
- For maintainance fluids, consider starting with D5 1/2NS for children >2 years; D51/4NS for children <2 years.
- Add *potassium* to maintainance fluids only after urine output confirmed.
- Adding additional base (*bicarbonate* or *acetate*) to the IVF is usually not necessary unless high ongoing losses (stool) or renal dysfunction exists.
- Do not adjust the serum Na^+ >10-15 mEq/L/day. If a patient's abnormality is greater than this, they must be admitted for volume and electrolyte correction over 24-48 hours.

Questions

1. A 6 week old infant arrives with her first time parents at 1am after several episodes of non-bilous emesis. She has a heart rate of 200 bpm, a fever of 39.0, and seems listless. What is the appropriate course of action?
   A. Try oral hydration and an anti-pyretic to resolve the tachycardia. Arrange follow-up with the pediatrician in the morning for gastroenteritis.
   B. Start an IV, give 10 ml/kg of normal *saline*, and discharge the patient when she can tolerate oral feeding. Diagnosis of gastroenteritis.
   C. Check her *glucose* immediately
   D. Initiate a work-up for a septic infant
   E. C and D

   Answer: E; this infant is septic until proven otherwise. Use caution in calling everything that vomits gastroenteritis.

2. A 4 year old child arrives with his family. They ate at the family reunion yesterday and all had vomiting and diarrhea for about 12 hours. He has persistent nausea and vomiting, but the diarrhea has stopped. He feels thirsty, but vomits after chugging his bottle of juice. He looks well with normal vital signs and a benign abdominal exam. How can you help?
   A. Initiate an IV and give repeated 20 ml/kg boluses
   B. Reassure parents that he will be OK, continue pushing fluids as much as they can, follow-up with their doctor as needed
   C. Slow down his intake to 30 ml every 15 minutes. Use a diluted sports drink or juice. Slowly increase the frequency of the feeding
   D. Use an anti-emetic such as ondansetron to aid in your oral rehydration
   E. C and/or D

   Answer: E, this child is not in shock, and does not need aggressive fluid resuscitation. Pushing fluids does not mean allowing a vomiting child to drink uncontrolled. Encourage parents to be creative in their "fluids." Use popcicles or other frozen treats, broth, or ice chips.

References

1. Practice parameter: the management of acute gastroenteritis in young children. American Academy of Pediatrics, Provisional Committee on Quality Improvement, Subcommittee on Acute Gastroenteritis. *Pediatrics* 1996 Mar; 97(3):424-35

Endocrine Emergencies

Giselle Zigari, MD
Department of Emergency Medicine
The University of Arizona

Diabetic Ketoacidosis

Critical Knowledge

- ABC's, supplemental O2
- 2 large bore IV's
- NPO
- Arterial line (shock, AMS, severe acidosis)
- Labs: immediate FSBS, ABG/VBG, UA w/osmolarity, serum electrolytes, serum *magnesium*, serum *calcium*, CBC w/ differential, serum osmolarity
- Assess dehydration
- Begin with isotonic fluids, 20 ml/kg bolus over 30-60 minutes
- Transition early to maintenance fluids for correction over 24-48 hours
- Administer *insulin*
- Empiric antibiotics – if infectious etiology thought to be present
- Monitor – ICU admission, pediatric endocrine consult

Background

- Definition: hyperglycemia, ketonemia, and acidosis due to untreated absolute (Type I) or relative (Type II) deficiency of *insulin*.
- Hyperglycemia: results from impaired uptake from lack of *insulin* or *insulin* insensitivity. Hyperosmotic serum pulls water out from cells leading to osmotic diuresis and causes hypovolemia. Hypovolemia leads to hypoperfusion, resulting in lactic acidosis.
- Ketonemia: *glucagon* is release to mobilize *glycogen* from liver for fuel for cells and also leads to lipolysis. Incomplete fatty acid oxidation leads to ketoacid formation: *Acetone*, *acetoacetate*, and *Beta-hydroxybutyrate*, of which only the two former are detected on UA. These (*acetone* and *acetoacetate*) increase as acidosis resolves, while *Beta-hydroxybutyrate* decreases. As acidosis worsens, the opposite is true. *THEREFORE: a UA may NOT reflect ketosis*.

- Acidosis: combination of ketosis and lactic acidosis
    - **A**nion **G**ap (**AG**) will be elevated (AG= Na^+ – (Cl + HCO3))
- Hyperkalemia may be seen initially even if *potassium* deficit exists
- As acidosis corrects, serum *potassium* levels will decrease
    - *Must correct severe *potassium* deficits before *insulin* administration*
    - Caused by an extracellular shift of K^+ as H^+ moves intracellularly due to excess (acidosis)
    - Also caused by decreased renal tubular excretion
    - EKG may show tall, peaked T waves
- Hypokalemia
    - May develop after *insulin* administration due to the correction of acidosis and the K^+ returning intracellularly.
    - Replace accordingly with IVF as described in Treatment Section.
    - EKG may show low T waves or U waves.
- Hyponatremia
    - Often observed as a dilutional effect of free water moving extracellularly due to the increased serum Osm from hyperglycemia.
    - Measurement of true serum Na^+ during hyperglycemia: serum Na^+ + 1.6 mEq per 100 mg/dL *glucose* over baseline *glucose* of 100.
- Hypophosphatemia
    - Results from acidosis, catabolism, *insulin* insufficiency, and osmotic diuresis
    - Often occurs during Tx of DKA

Complications

- Hypoglycemia
- Persistent acidosis
- Hypokalemia
- Cardiac dysrhythmias: hyperkalemia, hypokalemia, and/or hypocalcemia
- Pulmonary edema/ARDS: may be due to low plasma oncotic pressure and increased pulmonary capillary perfusion in combination with excessive crystalloid infusion
- Cerebral edema/herniation
    - Cause is considered multi-factorial
    - May occur from rapid correction of hyperglycemia and serum osmolarity

- Brain cells absorb *glucose* readily during hyperglycemia. If extracellular osmolarity drops rapidly due to correction of hyperglycemia, free water shifts intracellularly to the area of high *glucose* concentration within brain cells, resulting in edema.
- Occurs in 0.3-1% of all episodes of DKA
  - One third of cases leads to death
  - One third of cases lead to some type of neurological impairment
- High risk indicators
  - New-onset DM
  - Age <2 yrs
  - pH <7.1 or pc02 <20
  - Severe dehydration
  - Neuro changes
  - Cardiovascular instability
  - Rapid decline in blood *glucose*
  - Rehydration with hypotonic solutions
  - Use of *bicarbonate*
  - Rate of hydration >50 cc/kg/hr
- Usually occurs 4-24 hrs after therapy initiated
  - Patient appears to be improving chemically/clinically
  - 50% cases demonstrate neuro changes before collapse
  - HA, incontinence, behavior, papillary, BP, bradycardia, SZ, temp disregulation
  - Treatment: reduce ICP
  - ABC's
  - *Mannitol* (0.2-1 g/kg IV over 30 minutes)
  - Reduce fluids
  - Hyperventilation 5-10 breaths/minute over regular rate for age
  - *Glucocorticoids*

Differential Diagnosis

- *NOTE: classic symptoms are often absent in toddlers!*
- New onset diabetes: presenting symptoms
- Insidious

- 3P's: **P**olyuria, **P**olydipsia, **P**olyphagia
- Nausea/vomiting
- Abdominal pain
- Weight loss
- Fever
- Known diabetic: precipitating factors
- Missed *insulin* doses
- Infection/current illness *MOST FREQUENT CAUSE OF DKA* evaluate aggressively
- Drugs/alcohol
- Psychosocial stressors
- Poor compliance
- Trauma
- Pump failure
- DKA in non-diabetics
- *Salicylate* intoxication
- Pneumonia/asthma
- Head injury/CNS infection
- Dehydration
- Renal glucosuria
- Alcoholic ketoacidosis
- Large or small bowel obstruction
- Pancreatitis
- Gastroenteritis
- Pyloric stenosis
- What not to miss on initial presentation:
  - AMS without evidence of head trauma
  - Kussmaul respirations
  - *Acetone*/fruity odor on patient's breath - NOT everyone can detect this odor!
  - Don't forget the importance of a quick finger-stick!
  - *NOTE: sedation is contraindicated due to neuro and respiratory impairment. DO NOT GIVE *PHENERGAN**

Treatment

- ABC's
- Assess level of dehydration
    - Minimal: 1-2% (10-20 cc/kg)
        - Polydipsia
        - Mild oliguria
    - Mild: 3-5% (child-infant; 30-50 cc/kg)
        - Dry lips
        - Thick saliva
        - Decreased tears
        - Anterior fontanelle flat
        - Decreased urine output
    - Moderate: 6-9% (child-infant; 60-90 cc/kg)
        - Sunken eyes
        - Absent tears
        - Dry mucosa
        - Sunken fontanelle
        - Weak/rapid pulse
        - Decreased skin turgor
        - Cap refill >2 sec
        - Listless/irritable
        - Urine: dark, <1-2 cc/kg/hr, spc grav= 1.030, incr BUN
        - PH <7.3
    - Severe: 10-15% (child-infant; 100-150 cc/kg)
        - Limp and cold
        - Lethargy or coma
        - Acrocyanosis
        - Thready pulse
        - Grunting
        - Deep and rapid RR
        - Hypotension
        - Skin retracts >2 sec
        - Oliguria/anuria: spc grav >1.035

        - Cap refill >4 sec
        - Markedly incr. BUN
        - PH <7.0
- Fluid replacement: determine volume of fluid replacement
    - Deficit (% dehydration x body wt in kg) + maintenance given over 48 hours
    - *Approx. 1½ times maintenance fluids*
- Determine type of fluids to use: begin with 0.45 NS w/ 20 mEq KCl
- Order 2 bags of fluid and hang
    - ½ NS +/- K^+ and D10 ½ NS +/- K^+
    - ½ NS +/- K^+ will run at calculated rate
    - D10 ½ NS +/- K^+ may be titrated in while maintaining a constant rate, once *glucose* drops to 250 mg/dL.
- *Potassium*: *must be replaced prior to *insulin* administration*
    - Check EKG, urine output
    - K^+ must be >2.5 for *insulin* administration
    - Recheck K^+ levels hourly
    - Replacement
        - 2.5-3.5: add 40-60 mEq/L
        - 3.5-5.0: add 30-40 mEq/L
        - 5-5.5: add 20 mEq/L
        - >5.5: omit K from IVF
- Phosphorous
    - May drop with *insulin* therapy
    - Treat if there are cardiopulmonary effects (<0.5-1)
    - Avoid excessive replacement: may lead to hypocalcemic tetany
    - Use 50:50 mix of Kphos and KCl for K^+ replacement in the first 8 hours
- *Bicarbonate* *controversial*
    - May worsen cerebral acidosis and edema
    - Resultant alkalosis decreases O2 delivery to tissue due to a left-shifted O2 dissociation curve and hypokalemia due to intracellular shift of *potassium*
    - May be indicated in severe, refractory acidosis (pH <7.1 after 1 hr.

resuscitation) with evidence of decreased heart contractility or hypoventilation.
    - Consult PICU attending/endocrinologist
- *Insulin*
    - Begin drip at 0.1 units/kg/hr of regular *insulin*
        - 50 units in 500 cc= 0.1 unit/cc
        - *NOTE: flush IV tubing with *insulin* prior to administration as it binds to plastic tubing*
    - Continue until acidosis resolved
    - Begin SC *insulin* and D/C drip 30 min after SC dose
        - 0.1-0.25 units/kg q 6-8 hrs for new diabetic
        - Patient must be able to tolerate po's
        - Resume prior regimen in known diabetic
- *Glucose*
    - Should decrease 50-100 mg/dL/hr during *insulin* gtt
    - Want to maintain target blood sugar between 150-250
        - *Remember: hyperglycemia is not killing your patient! Treatment goal is to resolve acidosis that is the result of ketogenesis, not hyperglycemia!*
        - Acidosis reflects *insulin* deficiency: hyperglycemia reflects hydration status
    - Begin *glucose* infusion when blood *glucose* is about 300 mg/dL or if blood *glucose* drops more than 100 mg/dL/hr.
        - Titrate the contents of the D10 ½ NS bag with the currently running fluids while maintaining the overall rate at a constant.
        - *Insulin* dose should not be adjusted!
- ICU amission citeria
    - Aterial pH <7.3 or venous pH <7.25
    - AMS
    - Sever vomiting/dehydration
    - Gucose >600
- Monitoring: finger-sticks every hour
- Neuro checks every hour: *NOTE: this includes watching for bradycardia and hypertension, which are part of Cushing's Triad!*

- VBG every 2-4 hours
- Electrolytes every hour if unstable or every four hours if stable
- Urinalysis with each void to assess for ketones and *glucose*

Flow Sheet for Monitoring Diabetic Ketoacidosis							
Patient's Name ______________________							
Weight-Initial ____________ **After 24 hours** ____________							
Date **Hour**	0	1	2	3	4	5	6
General information							
Mental status*							
Temperature							
Pulse							
Respiration/depth†							
Blood pressure							
Serum *glucose* (mg/dL)							
Serum *ketones*							
Urinary *ketones*							
Electrolytes							
Serum *sodium* (mEq/L)							
Serum *potassium* (mEq/L)							
Serum *chloride* (mEq/L)							
Serum *bicarbonate* (mEq/L)							
Serum blood urea *nitrogen* (mg/dL)							
Effective osmolality: 2 (measured serum *sodium* [mEq/L]) + *glucose* (mg/dL)/18							
Anion gap (mEq/L)							
Arterial Blood Gases							
pH: venous (V); arterial (A)							
Pao2							
Paco2							
02 saturation							
Insulin							
Units in past hour							
Route							

Intake of Fluids/Metabolites							
0.45% *saline* (mL) in past hour							
0.9% *saline* (mL) in past hour							
5% *dextrose* (mL) in past hour							
Potassium chloride (mEq) in past hour							
Phosphate (mmol) in past hour							
Other							
Output							
Urine (mL)							
Other							
*--A=alert; D=drowsy; S=stuporous; C=comatose. †--D=deep; S=shallow; N=normal.							

FIGURE 3. A suggested flow sheet for monitoring response to therapy for diabetic ketoacidosis. (Pao2=partial pressure of oxygen; Paco2=partial pressure of arterial carbon dioxide)[7]

Questions

1. Which keto-acid is not detected by urinalysis?

   Answer: Beta-hydroxybutyrate (remember- the detectable ones may not be present in severe acidosis!)

2. Which electrolyte must be corrected prior to *insulin* administration?

   Answer: *Potassium*

3. What is the leading cause of mortality in DKA?

   Answer: Cerebral edema

References

1. Ellis EN. Concepts of fluid therapy in diabetic ketoacidosis and hyperosmolar hyperglycemic nonketotic coma. *Pediatr. Clin N Amer* 37:313-321, 1990.
2. Kitabchi AE, Wall BM. Diabetic ketosacidosis. *Med Clin N Amer* 79:9-37, 1995.
3. Keefer, JR. *The Harriet Lane Handbook: Endocrinology.* 15th Ed; 207-211. Eds. Siberry and Iannone. Mosby Inc. 2000
4. Porter. Pediatric Dehydration. *Ann Emerg Med* 41:196-205
5. Rosenbloom AL. *Intracerebral crises during treatment of diabetic ketoacidosis.* Diab Care 13:22-33, 1990.

6. Young GM. Pediatrics, *Diabetic Ketoacidosis*. www.emedicine.com/emerg/topic373.htm. March 27, 2006.
7. Adapted with permission from Kitabchi AE, Fisher JN, Murphy MB, Rumbak MJ. Diabetic ketoacidosis and the hyperglycemic hyperosmolar nonketotic state. In: Kahn CR, Weir GC, eds. Joslin's Diabetes mellitus. 13th ed. Baltimore: Williams & Wilkins, 1994:738-70.

Hypoglycemia

Critical Knowledge

- ABC's, supplemental O2
- 2 large bore IV's
- NPO
- Arterial line (shock, AMS, severe acidosis)
- Labs: immediate FSBS, ABG/VBG, UA w/ osmolarity, serum electrolytes, serum *magnesium*, serum *calcium*, CBC w/ differential, serum osmolarity
- *IMPORTANT* draw an extra heparinized tube and place on ice to be used for later testing by endocrinologist if necessary for lactate, pyruvate, beta-hydroxybutyrate, amino acid profile, acylcarnitine profile, toxicologic, and hormonal studies.
- Conscious patient without IV access taking PO's: 5-10 grams *glucose*
    - 5 g *glucose* tablet
    - 240 cc milk
    - 1 teaspoon granulated sugar (5 g/tsp)
- Unconscious patient with IV access
    - Peds:1-2 mL/kg of 25% *dextrose* solution
    - Infants/neonates: 2.5-5 mL/kg of 10% solution
- Unconscious patient without IV access OR failure to respond to *glucose*
    - *Glucagon* SC or IM
        - Children: 30 mcg/kg
        - Neonates: 50 mcg/kg
- Refractory hypoglycemia
- Empiric *steroids*: *hydrocortisone* 1-2 mg/kg IV q 6 hrs
- Suspected sulfonylurea overdose: *octreotide* 50-125 mcg SC

- Suspect hyperinsulinemic (endogenous *insulin*): *diazoxide*
  - Children/infants: 1-3 mg/kg q 8 hrs
  - Neonates: 3-5 mg/kg q 8 hrs
- Correct electrolytes
- Control seizures if refractory to *glucose* therapy
- Identify underlying cause and correct
- Appropriate surgical consult if endogenous cause suspected
- Severely affected neonates of <3 months not responsive to above therapy may require surgical exploration and subsequent sub-total pancreatectomy
- Monitor: PICU, endocrinology

Background

- Definition: blood *glucose* value <40 mg/dL; in neonates, <30 mg/dL for the first 24 hrs of life and <45 mg/dL thereafter.
- Whipple's triad (clinical definition): symptoms consistent with hypoglycemia, measured hypoglycemia, symptoms resolve as hypoglycemia resolves.
- Normal regulation of blood *glucose*: usually around 80-90 mg/dL
- *Glucose* increases transiently after meals to 120-140 mg/dL, should return to normal within 2 hrs post-prandial.
- *Insulin*: secreted when *glucose* is present and stimulates liver to store *glycogen* and muscles to uptake *glucose*. Excess is stored as fat. Inhibits lipolysis and *glycogen*olysis.
- *Glucagon*: increases blood *glucose* levels by stimulating liver to release *glucose* back into blood.
- Starvation: liver maintains *glucose* by gluconeogenesis (amino acid and glycerol break down) and ketosis. Hypothalamus causes *epinephrine* release by adrenals to stimulate further glucolysis from liver.
  - Prolonged hypoglycemia over hours-days will result in growth hormone and *cortisol* release to decrease *glucose* utilization by most cells of the body to preserve *glucose*.
- Newborn hypoglycemia: serum *glucose* declines after birth until 1-3 hrs, depleting liver *glycogen* stores rapidly. Gluconeogenesis via alanine results in rapid, spontaneous *glucose* return.
- Older infants/children *glucose* homeostasis: glycogenolysis in immediate postfeeding period and gluconeogenesis several hours after meals.

- In diabetic patients: long-standing type I
  - Develop loss of *glucagon* secretion in response to hypoglycemia
  - *Epinephrine* is release at a lower *glucose* threshold.
  - Hypoglycemic unawareness = loss of warning symptoms of hypoglycemia that previously prompted the patient to eat
- Septic, liver/renal failure patients: cause is multi-factorial due to deficient *cortisol* or thyroid hormone.
- Recurrent, spontaneous hypoglycemia: hyperinsulinism due to insulinoma, iatrogenic insulin or sulfonylurea drug use, insulin autoantibodies, or tumors
- Hyperinsulinism
  - Onset = birth - 18 months
  - Inappropriately elevated *insulin* at time of hypoglycemia
  - Transient neonatal hyperinsulinism in macrosomic infants of diabetic mothers
  - Due to diminished *glucagon* secretion and inhibited endogenous *glucose* production.
  - Manifests as increasing demands for feeding, intermittent lethargy, jitteriness, and frank seizures.
- Ketotic hypoglycemia
  - Observed in children younger than 5 years who usually become symptomatic after an overnight or prolonged fast, especially with illness and poor oral intake.
  - Children often present inexplicably lethargic or frankly comatose, having only marked hypoglycemia with ketonuria

Differential Diagnosis

Decreased Availability of *Glucose*	Increased use of *Glucose*	Diminished Availability of Alternative Fuels	Unknown or Complex Mechanisms
Decreased intake: fasting, malnutrition, illness	Hyperinsulinism: islet cell adenoma or hyperplasia, ingestion of oral hypoglycemic agents, *insulin* therapy, infants of diabetic mothers, Beckwith Wiedman Syndrome	Decreased or absent fat stores	Sepsis, shock, burns, cardiogenic shock, ARDS
Decreased absorption: acute diarrhea	Large tumors: Wilm's tumor, neuroblastoma	Inability to oxidize fats: enzymatic defects in fatty acid oxidation	Reye's Syndrome, hepatitis, cirrhosis, hepatoma
Inadequate *glycogen* reserves: defects in *glycogen*olytic pathway enzymes	Hyperthermia		Ingestions: *salicylate*, *ethanol*, *isoniazid*, *propanolol*, *pentamidine*, *quinine*, *disopyramide*, rat poison
Inability to mobilize *glycogen*: *glucagon* deficiency.	Polycythemia		Adrenal insufficiency
Ineffective gluconeogenesis: defects in enzymes of gluconeogenic pathway	Growth hormone deficiency		Hypothyroidism, hypopituitarism

- What not to miss: signs and symptoms of hypoglycemia re NONSPECIFIC and are often OVERLOOKED
  - Adrenergic symptoms
    - Palpitations
    - Anxiety
    - Tremulousness
    - Hunger
    - Sweating
  - Neurologic symptoms
    - Irritability
    - Headache
    - Fatigue
    - Confusion
    - Seizure
    - Unconsciousness

Treatment

- Treat initial hypoglycemia as presented above
- Maintain blood *glucose* via infusion with D10W at 1½ times maintenance (6-8 mg/kg/min)
- Goal is to maintain blood sugar higher than 70 mg/dL.
- Admission criteria
  - *ANY child with documented hypoglycemia NOT secondary to *insulin* therapy*
  - Continued or recurrent altered mental status
  - Decreasing serial *glucose* levels despite *glucose* therapy
  - Large doses of *glucose* required during replacement therapy
  - Known/suspected history of massive *insulin* or *sufonylurea* overdose
  - Severe underlying disease: sepsis, renal/hepatic failure, endocrine deficiency
  - No responsible caregiver to monitor blood *glucose* q 3 hrs at home and give repeated feedings.

Questions

1. What is normal, fasting blood sugar?

   Answer: 80-90 mg/dL

2. What does *glucagon* do in blood sugar homeostasis?

   Answer: Increases blood *glucose* levels by stimulating liver to release *glucose* back into blood.

3. At what age is surgical consultation considered in cases of hypoglycemia?

   Answer: Infants <3 months not responsive to *glucose* therapy.

4. What does exploratory surgery hope to find?

   Answer: Pancreatic mass (excessive beta cells excreting *insulin*)

References

1. Agus, MSD. Textbook of Pediatric Emergency Medicine: *Endocrine Emergencies- Hypoglycemia*. 5th Ed. Ed's Fleisher GR, et al. Lippincott Williams and Wilkins, Philadelphia, 2001.
2. Cranmer, H. Pediatric Hypoglycemia. www.emedicine.com/emerg/topic384.htm. March 15, 2005.
3. Shah, I. *Hypoglycemia*. Pediatric Oncall. Jan 7, 2006.www.pediatriconcall.com.

Hypocalcemic Crisis

Critical Knowledge

- ABC's
- IV
- 02
- Monitor and 12-lead EKG (long Q-T)
- Labs
  - Stat: *calcium*, *phosphorus*, *magnesium*, *albumin*, *ionized calcium*
  - Total protein, BUN/*creatinine*, parathyroid hormone, pH, urine *calcium/phosphorous/mag*
- Recognize frank tetany, laryngospasm, seizures, and treat

Background

- Total *calcium* level reflects bound and unbound (ionized) *calcium*
- Ionized component is physiologically active
  - Affected by *albumin* level, blood pH, serum *phosphate* and serum *magnesium*.
  - Reduced by anything that may bind *calcium*: citrate from blood transfusions or free fatty acids from TPN
- Corrected serum *calcium* level in hypoalbuminemia
- (0.8 x (normal albumin-patient *albumin*)) + Ca
- CNS effects
  - Hypocalcemia decreases the threshold of neuronal excitability, allowing repetitive responses from a single stimulus
  - Affects both motor and sensory nerves
- Tetany
  - Hypocalcemia should depress muscular excitability by impeding acetylcholine release at neuromuscular junction.
  - Results from an override of inhibitory muscle contraction and sensitive neuronal excitability.
- *Calcium* homeostasis
- Vitamin D (1,25(OH)2D3)
  - Raises serum *calcium* by absorbing *calcium* and *phosphorous* from the gut
  - Enhances PTH-dependent *calcium* mobilization from bone
  - Promotes renal conservation of *calcium*.
- Parathyroid hormone
  - Increases *calcium* resorption from bone
  - Increases renal *phosphorous* excretion and decreases renal *calcium* excretion
  - Enhances conversion of Vitamin D to active form
- *ERGO: hypocalcemia results from a defect/deficiency in the above mentioned regulatory pathways
  - Vitamin D or PTH deficiency
  - End-organ resistance to these hormones due to lack of receptors or abnormal receptor binding

Differential Diagnosis

- *DO NOT MISS*: life-threatening manifestations
- Tetany
- Seizure
- Laryngospasm/stridor
- Prolonged QT, conduction abnormalities with bradycardia

Early/Neonatal (1-3 days)	Late Neonatal (3d- 6 wks)	Infancy/Childhood
Prematurity: poor intake, decreased Vit D responsiveness, increased calcitonin, hypoalbuminemia	Idiopathic hypoparathyroidism: transient vs. permanent	Hypoparathyroidism: autoimmune, post-surgical/post-irradiation, hypomagnesemia, pseudo-hypoparathyroidism (PTH receptor defect), infiltration (iron overload- Wilson's dz, hemosiderosis, thalassemia)
Hypoxic encephalopathy/ birth asphyxia: delayed feeds, incr. calcitonin, incr phosphate, alkali therapy	Maternal hypercalcemia	Hyperphosphatemia: improper formula, inappropriate use of phos-containing enemas, loading in TPN, renal failure
IUGR	Congenital Aplasia: DiGeorge Syndrome, Velo-Cardio-Facial Syndrome	Chelation, blood transfusions
Exchange transfusion (citrate load)	Cow's milk tetany: due to high phosphate load with cow's milk	Acute severe illness; Malabsorption Syndromes
Infant of diabetic mother	Chronic diarrhea: *calcium/magnesium* malabsorption, alkaline Tx for acidosis, renal losses of *calcium/ magnesium*	Pancreatitis

Early/Neonatal (1-3 days)	Late Neonatal (3d- 6 wks)	Infancy/Childhood
Magnesium deficiency	Hypomagnesemia	Rickets; "Hungry Bone Syndrome" after Tx of rickets
	Severe infantile osteopetrosis	Alkalosis: respiratory or metabolic

Treatment

- Acute treatment of symptomatic hypocalcemia
    - 0.5-1 mL/kg 10% *calcium gluconate* IV over 3-5 minutes
    - Up to 2mL /kg IV over 20 minutes.
    - Can repeat every 6-8 hours
- *NOTE: patient must remain on cardiac monitor and therapy stopped if HR <60*
- Therapy may be added to IV solution once symptoms relieved or administered orally
- Maintenance infusion
    - <2 yrs= 8 mL/kg/day 10% *calcium gluconate*
    - >2 yrs= 5 mgL/kg/day 10% *calcium gluconate*
- *NOTE: precautions for IV *calcium**
    - Ensure dilute solution to minimize risk of burn
    - Ensure proper IV flow to avoid SC tissue burn
    - Never mix with fluids containing *phosphate* or *bicarb*
    - Monitor serum *calcium* frequently
- Acute correction of hypomagenesemia (Mg <1.5 mg/dL)
- If thought to be the cause of hypocalcemia, administer *magnesium* first, IM route
- Treat if hypocalcemia refractory to *calcium* supplementation.
- 0.2 mL/kg IM of 50% Mg *sulfate*. May repeat q 8-12 hrs.
- Maintenance: begin 250-500 mg po QID when possible. IV *magnesium* excreted rapidly.
- Significant hyperphosphatemia: correct before *calcium* replacement to prevent soft tissue calcification.

- Give phosphate binders: *calcium carbonate, aluminum hydroxide*
- For cell lysis: NS boluses and IV *mannitol*
- In renal failure: dialysis
- Admission criteria
  - Any newborn infant with hypocalcemia should be monitored in the NICU.
  - Any child with symptomatic hypocalcemia should be admitted to the hospital unless the diagnosis is hyperventilation

Questions

1. What two cardiac dysrrhythmias are seen with hypocalcemia?

   Answer: Prolong Q-T, bradycardia

2. What electrolyte disturbance should be considered if hypocalcemia is refractory to therapy?

   Answer: Hypomagnesemia

3. What liver function abnormality must be considered with low serum *calcium* levels?

   Answer: Hypoalbuminemia

References

1. Agus, SD. Textbook of Pediatric Emergency Medicine: *Endocrine Emergencies- Hypocalcemia*. 5th Ed. Ed's Fleisher GR, et al. Lippincott Williams and Wilkins, Philadelphia, 2001.
2. Choukair, MK. *The Harriet Lane Handbook: Fluids and Electolytes*. 15th Ed; 243-246. Eds. Siberry and Iannone. Mosby Inc. 2000.
3. Muir, A. *Care of children with Hypocalcemic crisis*. http://www.mcg.edu/pediatrics/pedsendo/hypocalcemia.htm. Feb. 27, 2004.
4. Singhal A, Campbell DE. *Pediatric Hypocalcemia*. http://www.emedicine.com/ped/topic1111.htm. Sept. 14, 2006.

Adrenal Crisis

Critical Knowledge

- ABCD's (D= dextrose level), O_2
- IV
- Monitor
- Labs: electrolytes, fasting blood sugar, serum ACTH, plasma renin activity, serum *cortisol*, serum *aldosterone*
- Recognize diagnosis by hypoglycemia, hyponatremia, hyperkalemia, metabolic acidosis, shock, and ambiguous genitalia
- Immediate volume expansion with 20 mL/kg IV NS boluses
- Maintain blood sugar with 10% dextrose
- Intravenous *hydrocortisone*
- Sepsis workup for precipitating cause and empiric antibiotics if suspected

Background

- Definition: adrenal cortex fails to produce enough *glucocorticoid* and *mineralocorticoid* in response to stress
- May be primary: adrenal disorder
- Secondary: hypothalamic-pituitary disorder
- *Mineralocorticoids/aldosterone*
    - Maintain salt and water homeostasis
    - Promotes salt resorption in distal renal tubules and collecting ducts
    - Regulated by rennin-angiotensin system, therefore, not deficient in secondary adrenal insufficiency
- *Glucocorticoids/cortisol*
    - Important hormone in mounting a response to stress, such as infection, surgery, or trauma and promotes gluconeogenesis and protein and fat breakdown
    - Release is stimulated by **C**orticotropin **R**eleasing **H**ormone (**CRH**) from the hypothalamus to pituitary and from ACTH from the pituitary to the adrenals
    - Low levels of *cortisol* stimulate ACTH release, ergo ACTH levels will be high in primary adrenal insufficiency

- Congenital adrenal hyperplasia: 90% of all cases due to 21-hydroxylase deficiency
  - Enzyme necessary for *cortisol* and *aldosterone* production
  - ACTH increases, precursors of *cortisol/aldosterone* accumulate
  - Androgen production is increased due to shunting of the *cortisol/aldosterone* production pathway.
    - Females virilized in utero, born with ambiguous genitalia, and often identified at birth
    - Enlarged clitoris and fusion of labial folds
    - Males often have normal genitalia development, so more likely to present with salt-wasting crisis in infancy or demonstrate precocious puberty
    - Undervirilized males: small phallus, hypospadias, gonads in inguinal canals
    - Hyperpigmentation of labioscrotal folds and nipples
- Adrenal crisis often presents at 2-5 weeks of age
  - Symptoms often insidious: poor feeding, lack of weight gain, lethargy, irritability, vomiting
  - Hyponatremia: due to lack of *aldosterone* and inability to spare *sodium* ("salt-wasting")
  - Hypoglycemia: may be due to lack of *cortisol* and/or reduced caloric intake during acute illness
  - Hyperkalemia
    - Serum levels often between 6-12 mEq /L without EKG changes
    - May appear to be within normal limits if vomiting and diarrhea have occurred.
  - Metabolic acidosis
    - Reflected by low bicarb
    - Due to retention of hydrogen ions in exchange for *sodium* loss

Differential Diagnosis

Primary Adrenal Insufficiency	Secondary Adrenal Insufficiency
Hereditary: congenital adrenal hyperplasia, adrenoleukodystrophy, mineralocorticoid deficiency, Refsum dz, Wolman dz	Iatrogenic: inadequte glucocorticoid administration, withdrawl from glucocorticoid therapy
Autoimmune: Addison's, IDDM, thyroiditis	Tumors: pituitary or hypothalamic
Infection: tuberculosis, meningococcal septicemia, systemic fungal infections, HIV	CNS surgery or irradiation
Adrenal hemorrhage	Structural abnormalities: septooptic dysplasia
Meds that increase steroid metabolism: *rifampin*, *phenytoin*, *phenobarbitol*	Congenital hypopituitarism
Meds that decrease steroid synthesis: *etomidate*, *ketoconazole*	Isolated ACTH deficiency

Treatment

- Immediate volume expansion with 20 mL/kg IV NS
- Immediate *hydrocortisone* IV
  - ▶ <3 yrs= 25 mg
  - ▶ 3-12 yrs= 50 mg
  - ▶ >12 yrs= 100 mg
  - ▶ Subsequent= 50 mg/m2/24 hrs. IV or q 6 hrs
- Hyperkalemia
- Correct if cardiac arrhythmias present
  - ▶ 10% *calcium gluconate*: 1 mL/kg IV over 3-5 min
  - ▶ *Kayexalate*: 1-2 mg/kg po (if taking po's)
  - ▶ *Insulin*: 0.1 units/kg IV with 2 mL/kg of 25% *glucose* 1-2 mEq/kg IV
  - ▶ *Bicarb*: 1-2 mEq/kg IV over 5-10 min
- NOTE: flush line after giving *calcium gluconate*, as *bicarb* not compatible.
- Identify and treat any precipitating cause: infection and/or trauma

- Long-term *mineralocorticoid* replacement
  - 0.05-0.2 mg/day *fludrocortisone* acetate PO
  - NOTE: initial *hydrocortisone* at 50 mg/m2 /day will supply initial maintenance amount of necessary *mineralocorticoid*
- Admit PICU
- Close hydration and blood sugar monitoring
- Check electrolytes q 2-4 hrs
- Replace 50% fluid deficit in first 8 hrs with NS and 10% *dextrose* and remainder over next 24 hrs.

Questions

1. What is the electrolyte disturbances encountered in acute adrenal crisis?

   Answer: Hyponatremia, hypoglycemia, hyperkalemia, metabolic acidosis
2. What immediate intervention will resolve most of these abnormalities?

   Answer: Immediate fluid resuscitation
3. What physical manifestations might be observed in the neonate that would suggest the diagnosis of congenital adrenal hyperplasia?

   Answer: Ambiguous genitalia in females, hypospadias, hyperpigmented nipples, and undescended testes in males

References

1. Agus, SD. Textbook of Pediatric Emergency Medicine: *Endocrine Emergencies-Acute Adrenal Insufficiency.* 5th Ed.:97; 1176-1180. Ed's Fleisher GR, et al. Lippincott Williams and Wilkins, Philadelphia, 2001
2. Keefer, JR. *The Harriet Lane Handbook: Endocrinology.* 15th Ed.:10; 209-211. Eds. Siberry and Iannone. Mosby Inc. 2000
3. Macdougall, P. *Adrenal Insufficiency: an Approach.* Chidren's & Women's Health centre of British Columbia. http://www.cw.bc.ca/pediatricresidents/aiapprch.asp, 1997.
4. Muir, A. *Management of Children with an adrenal crisis.*
5. http://www.mcg.edu/pediatrics/pedsendo/adrenal.htm. Feb 27, 2004.

The Febrile Child

Ben A. Leeson, MD
Department of Emergency Medicine
The University of Arizona
Kimberly A. B. Leeson, MD
Department of Emergency Medicine
The University of Arizona

Critical Knowledge

- Fever is defined as a temperature above 38.0° C (100.4° F)
- Fevers reported by guardians should be considered true fevers
- Acute otitis media should never be considered a source for fever
- ALL neonates (<28 days) with fever should be admitted and have a full sepsis workup
- Fever without localized source algorithms have been established to be used for "low risk" infants and are not meant for use on "high risk" infants

Background

A fever is defined as a temperature above 38.0° C (100.4° F) and may be an indication of a serious bacterial infection. Workup and treatment depends on many factors including the child's age, appearance, risk factors for serious infections, and availability of follow up.

Newborns and children up to the age of 3 years old are at relatively increased risk for bacteremia and serious infections. The risk decreases with age with the highest incidence during the first 3 months of life. Because of this, the pediatric patient with a fever is usually grouped by age: the neonatal period (28 days or less), 1-3 months, 3 months and older.

- Fever may account for up to 1/2 of ED pediatric visits
- A life threatening event occurs in up to 1% of children presenting with fever
- While most illnesses in young children are viral in nature, as many as 5% without an obvious source will have bacteremia
- Infants often present with non-specific symptoms with no localizing signs – assessment of a child's behavior and appearance often provide the most clues to illness severity
- The degree of fever, rapidity of rise or response to antipyretics do not predict seriousness of illness
- Performing a thorough history and physical are vital

- Any child under 3 who appears ill requires a workup and admission, regardless of whether a fever exists or not

Differential Diagnosis

- Infectious (etiologic agent varies by age)
  - Meningitis
  - Pyelonephritis
  - Bacterial or viral pneumonia
  - Otitis media
  - Localized skin infections (i.e., cellulitis/abscess)
  - Osteomyelitis
  - Oral infections such as pharyngitis from S. pyogenes and viral herpetic gingivostomatits
  - Generalized viral illness
- Noninfectious
  - High external temperature (especially in warmer months)
  - Overbundling children in cooler months (controversial)
  - Malignancy
  - Rheumatologic disease
  - Recent vaccination (especially with DTaP and MMR)
  - Ingestion including *aspirin* and anticholinergics (especially in toddler group)

Diagnostics and ED Treatment

- Establish "low risk" or "high risk"
  - Criteria for low risk
    - Previously healthy infants
    - Non-toxic appearance without an obvious focal bacterial infection
    - UA (negative nitrites and less than 10 wbc/hpf)
    - Serum WBC count between 5,000 and 15,000
    - Negative CSF gram stain and less than 8 WBC/mm3
    - Stool negative and few WBCs in stool if diarrhea is present
    - No pulmonary infiltrate if CXR is obtained
    - A complete exam looking for signs of infection must be performed.
  - Skin (classic rashes, cellulitis, osler nodes, etc.)

- ▸ HEENT (pharyngitis, peritonsillar abscess, lymphadenitis, etc.)
- ▸ Cardiovascular (new murmur or rub)
- ▸ Respiratory (tachypnea, wheezing, stridor)
- ▸ Abdomen (appendicitis or other surgical emergency)
- ▸ Neurologic (behavior, meningeal signs)
- ▸ Genitourinary
- ▸ Musculoskeletal (septic joint, osteomyelitis)

- Full sepsis workups include a CBC, blood culture, catheterized urinalysis and lumbar puncture.
- Include a chest radiograph if respiratory signs or symptoms are present (focal findings, tachypnea, SaO_2 <95%).
- Include rapid RSV/influenza and viral cultures if suspect
- Antipyretic (*acetaminophen* 15 mg/kg)
- Hospital admission versus outpatient management (see Figure 1)

Typical Antibiotic Coverage: Do Not Delay Administration in ill Appearing Patients

- Less than 2 months old: *ampicillin* 200 mg/kg/day (dosed every 6 hours) and *cefotaxime* 150 mg/kg/day (dosed every 8 hours) or *gentamycin* (loading dose based on age, typically 2.5 mg/kg/dose)
- Over two months old: third generation *cephalosporin* (*ceftriaxone* is often used for outpatient management based on its' once a day dosing regiment)
- Consider *vancomycin* for all ill appearing patients (*pneumococcal* antibiotic resistance has been rising and varies by region)

Neonatal Fever (Birth-1 Month of Age)

During the neonatal period (28 days or less), children are at a particularly high risk of developing emergent infections that require acute treatment. A complete sepsis workup including a lumbar puncture is indicated in this age group. Timely initiation of antibiotics is a top priority.

Fever without a Localizing Source in "Low Risk" Children 1-3 Months of Age

If the infant appears ill, the above full septic workup and conservative treatment should be initiated. High-risk patients in this age group include patients who have a history of prematurity, prolonged NICU stays, complicated births and congenital heart disease. Low risk patients may be treated on an outpatient basis. (see Figure 1)

In addition to appearing well and having a negative workup, the infant must have a stable home environment with reliable parents and close follow up must be ensured before a child in this age group can be discharged.

Fever without a Localizing Source in "Low Risk" Children 3-36 Months of Age

For children in this age group, management is based on the localizing signs and symptoms and the height of the temperature. Children with a source of the fever (pneumonia, urinary tract infection, etc.) should be treated accordingly and disposition depends on the severity of illness, ability to maintain hydration and tolerate oral medications and availability of close follow up.

The incidence of occult bacteremia has dramatically decreased since the introduction of the **HIB** (**H** **I**nfluenzae type **B**) and conjugated *pneumococcal* vaccines. For children less than 1 year of age with a fever of unknown origin greater than 39.0, most physicians will obtain both blood and urine for analysis and culture. Empiric antibiotics should be reserved for ill-appearing children and high-risk patients.

Fever without a Localizing Source in "Low Risk" Children Over 36 Months of Age

History and physical exam are both more reliable in children greater than 36 months. Working up children in this age group will focus on the presenting signs and symptoms. Treatment depends largely on the suspected etiology and can vary from supportive therapy to rescucitation and admission.

Questions

1. All of the following are true EXCEPT
    A. Fever in a child, especially less than 3 months of age, may be an indication of a serious bacterial infection
    B. Acute otitis media can be considered a source of fever in the neonate and full septic workup not performed
    C. Full septic workup includes blood culture, catheterized urine, and lumbar puncture
    D. Risk for serious bacterial infection decreases with age

    Answer: B

2. A 6 week old well-appearing infant is brought to the emergency department for fever. The child is found to have a temperature of 38.5 rectally. This patient may be discharged if

A. WBC between 5,000-15,000
B. 24 hour follow up can be arranged
C. Previously healthy
D. Negative CSF gram stain
E. Reliable parents
F. All of the above must be true

Answer: F

Figure 1 - Suggested Algorithm for Children with Fever

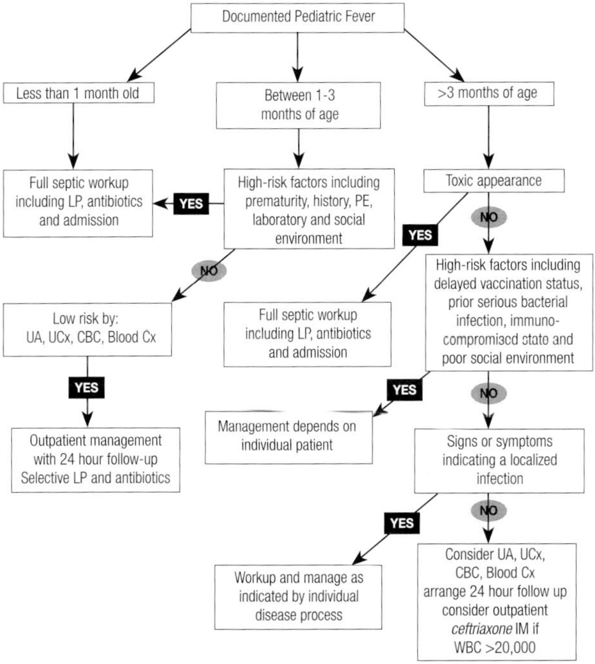

References

1. Royal Children's Hospital Clinical Practice Guidelines, www.rch.org.au/clinicalguide
2. www.emedicine.com/PED/topic2698.htm (accessed June 15, 2007)
3. www.emedicine.com/PED/topic3009.htm (accessed June 15, 2007)
4. www.emedicine.com/PED/topic2700.htm (accessed June 15, 2007)
5. ACEP: Clinical policy for children younger than three years presenting to the emergency department with fever. ACEP Clinical Policies Committee. *Ann Emerg Med* 2003 Oct; 42 (4): 530-545
6. Emergency Medicine, A Comprehensive Study Guide, 5th edition, *Tintinalli*, Kelen, Stapczynski pg 802-805

Fluid Resuscitation

Larry DeLuca, EdD, MD
Department of Emergency Medicine
The University of Arizona

Background

- Hypovolemia is the most common cause of shock in children. Hypovolemia can be absolute (as in hemorrhage or dehydration from diarrhea or vomiting) or relative (as in sepsis, where vasodilation increases the size of the "tank").
- Hypovolemia can span a range of severities, from mild dehydration to circulatory collapse. Here are some useful markers to determine the severity of hypovolemia.

	Mild Dehydration	Compensated Shock	Decompensated Shock	Circulatory Collapse
Heart Rate	Normal or slightly tachycardic	Slight tachycardia	Moderate tachycardia	Severe tachycardia
Blood Pressure	Normal	Low-normal	Low	Low or absent
Capillary Refill	<2 seconds	>2 seconds	>3 seconds	>5 seconds
Pulses	Strong	Proximal strong, distal weak	Proximal weak, distal absent	Proximal weak or absent
Mental Status	Normal	Irritable or confused	Agitated or lethargic	Obtunded or comatose

Adapted from American College of Surgeons' Committee on Trauma, from Advanced Trauma Life Support for Doctors (ATLS) Student Manual, 2004 (7th Edition). American College of Surgeons.

- Hypovolemia can have many causes, from increased insensible losses during fever to hemorrhage from trauma to vomiting and diarrhea. However, regardless of the cause of the hypovolemia, the most important initial intervention for hypovolemia from any cause is crystalloid fluid resuscitation.

Critical Knowledge

- Capillary refill by itself is not always reliable
    1. Cold extremities can simulate shock
- Pay close attention to mental status
    1. As shock evolves, blood is shunted to the heart and brain at the expense of the periphery
    2. Agitation suggests decreasing cerebral perfusion and impending decompensation
- Hypotension in children is an ominous sign
    1. Unlike adults, children will maintain a near-normal blood pressure until they are close to cardiopulmonary collapse
- Urinary output is not useful to guide initial resuscitation, but can help assess adequacy of resuscitation over time
    1. Normal urinary output is 0.5-1 mL/kg/hr
    2. Neonates and infants have less urinary concentrating capability, and may not conserve water as readily as older children and adults
    3. Be sure to ask parents or caregivers about the number of wet diapers a child has produced compared to normal
    4. Be sure that this represents urinary output and not volume losses from diarrhea
- One of the most common causes of **P**ulseless **E**lectrical **A**ctivity (**PEA**) "cardiac arrest" is profound hypovolemia
- One or more fluid boluses promptly administered can be lifesaving!

Normal Heart Rates Vary by Age

- Newborn to 3 months – mean 140 (awake 85-205; asleep 80-160)
- 3 months to 2 years – mean 130 (awake 100-190; asleep 75-160)
- 2 years to 10 years – mean 80 (awake 60-140; asleep 60-90)
- 10 years and over – mean 75 (awake 60-100; asleep 50-90)

Normal and Low-Normal Systolic Blood Pressure Vary by Age

- For children ages 1 to 10
    - Normal SBP = 90 mm Hg + (age * 2) mm Hg
    - Low-normal SBP = 70 mm Hg + (age * 2) mm Hg
    - For children 10 years and over, low-normal is approximately 90 mm Hg

Critical Concepts

There are many causes for hypovolemia. Fluid resuscitation is not definitive care, but part of patient stabilization. An important part of a successful resuscitation is identifying the factors that led to the need for fluid resuscitation and addressing them. For example, prompt administration of crystalloid fluids and blood products to a trauma patient will do little good if bleeding cannot be stopped. Aggressively search for and treat the causes of hypovolemia.

There are many different IV fluids available, and during resuscitation and ongoing therapy you may change from one fluid to another (for example, from crystalloid to packed red blood cells) as the resuscitation progresses, depending upon the patient's illness and the specifics of their clinical situation. For initial resuscitation, the fluid of choice is isotonic crystalloid (either normal *saline* (0.9%) or *Lactated Ringer's* Solution) given in boluses of 20 mL/kg. Once the patient is stabilized, IV fluid therapy can be adjusted based upon laboratory results (such as hematocrit or electrolyte status) and tailored to the patient's specific needs.

Fluid resuscitation does not need to occur via the IV route. For children who can tolerate oral intake, but have lost volume due to fever or diarrhea, oral rehydration may be an acceptable and convienent alternative. It is important to ensure that the child can consume adequate amounts of fluid orally, or dehydration and hypovolemia will worsen. It is also important to use a balanced electrolyte solution (such as Pedialyte) for oral fluid replacement. Replacing fluid losses with water only can result in hyponatremia and other electrolyte disturbances.

In critically ill children, consider **I**ntra**O**sseus (**IO**) access early on. After 3 unsuccessful attempts or 90 seconds of attempted IV access in a child with shock, place an IO line. The most common place for inserting an IO line is on the flat portion of the tibia that is 1 cm below and 1 cm medial to the tibial tuberosity. However, the distal femur, distal tibia, or iliac crest can also be used. Some areas are more likely for success depending on the age of the child. IO access can allow the infusion of any fluid, medication, or blood product, often at rates that exceed those of small-bore peripheral IV's.

- Be sure to address ongoing fluid needs as well as volume deficits
- The 4:2:1 rule is a convenient way to calculate pediatric maintenance IV rates
  - 4 mL /kg/hr for the first 10 kg of body weight +
  - 2 mL/kg /hr for the next 10 kg of body weight +
  - 1 mL/kg/hr for the remaining kg of body weight

*Example: a 25 kg child will require a maintenance rate of (4 * 10) + (2 * 10) + (1 * 5) = 65 mL/hr.*

Critical Concepts – IV Fluid Choices for Initial Resuscitation

There are an enormous number of IV fluid formulations, some standard, and some proprietary. Common prepared IV fluids vary in the amount of electrolytes, *glucose*, and free water, and other additives they contain. Patients with normal cardiopulmonary and renal function allow more flexibility in the IV fluids they receive, as they can more effectively filter what they do not need and excrete it. Patients who are oliguric, anuric, or who have compromised cardiorespiratory function will require more precise fluid selection and management (much of which is beyond the scope of this chapter).

For initial resuscitation, crystalloid fluids are the mainstay in modern practice, best exemplified by normal *saline* and *Lactated Ringer's*. These fluids are isotonic, providing about the same osmolality as intra- and extra-cellular fluid under normal conditions. They contain only electrolytes (no proteins or *glucose*). In theory they should provide minimal shifting of water across fluid compartments. Normal *saline* is a 0.9% solution of *sodium chloride* in water. The amount of *sodium* is in excess to that in blood – 154 mEq/L. In contast, *Lactated Ringer's* contains *sodium*, *chloride*, *potassium*, *calcium*, and lactate in amounts closer to that of serum levels of these electrolytes.

While technically still crystalloid solutions, the dextrose-containing solutions such as D5, D10, etc., are not used in initial resuscitation. These solutions provide "free water" - after the dextrose is metabolized, solute-free water remains.

Colloid solutions get their tonicity from albumin or synthetic polymers. It has been demonstrated that crystalloid solutions rapidly redistribute themselves in the body's various fluid compartments. For example, within several hours approximately 2/3 of infused normal *saline* is extra-vascular. Colloid solutions were supposed to solve this problem. However, even the larger colloid particles can and do migrate out of the vasculature, and having done so can occasionally worsen conditions such as peripheral edema. Colloid solutions are also more expensive, and also have allergenic potential. For all these reasons, crystalloid solutions have become the preferred solutions for initial resuscitation.

Critical Concepts – IV Fluid Choices for Fluid Maintenance

While isotonic crystalloids are ideal for initial resuscitation, they are poorly suited for maintenance. This is because they contain relatively large amounts of electrolytes, many crystalloids contain no *glucose*, and no free water. Infusing normal *saline* for many days, for example, can lead to *sodium* overload (and consequent fluid retention).

The most common maintenance IV fluids are D5 ½ NS, and D10 ¼ NS for infants up to 6 months. These fluids contain ½ (or ¼, respectively) as much *saline* as NS, avoiding the problem of over administration of *saline*. The solutions are hypotonic (providing some free water) and they contain dextrose (to help meet the body's *glucose* needs and reduce catabolism). The lower-*sodium* content of D10 ¼ NS is used with infants in the first 6 months of life because their renal concentrating ability is reduced compared to older children and adults.

Frequently, 10-20 mEq of *potassium* is added to each liter of maintenance fluid for patients with normal renal function.

Critical Concepts – Blood and Blood Products in Resuscitation

Blood transfusions may be required for any of a number of reasons in critically ill children, from blood loss through hemorrhage to acquired coagulopathy. While a detailed discussion of transfusion medicine is beyond the scope of this chapter, there are a few key concepts that can help guide you in selecting blood products.

While transfusion of blood products can provide life-saving benefits to patients, there is a substantial risk of infusing blood products compared to other IV fluids. While the HIV epidemic has caused people to be concerned with the safety of transfusions from a blood-borne disease perspective, these are not the only dangers faced by transfusion recipients. Allergic reactions are not uncommon, and can range from mild itching to full-blown anaphylaxis. Transfusion reactions from mistyped or non-cross-matched blood can result in hemolysis, renal failure, and death. Always take care when writing orders for blood transfusions and remember the simple maxim: *the most common cause of transfusion-related death is simple human error.*

There are Three Main Blood Products Commonly Used in Transfusion

- **Packed red blood cells** are cells separated from plasma by centrifugation. They can be filtered further to remove white cells (leukoreduction), which helps reduce both disease transmission and immune-mediated transfusion reactions. Use packed red blood cells to replace blood lost in trauma if a patient fails to respond to initial crystalloid resuscitation, or for profound and symptomatic anemia.
- **Plasma** (most commonly supplied as **F**resh **F**rozen **P**lasma (**FFP**)) contains plasma proteins, clotting factors, *albumin*, and other substances – all but the cellular components of blood. It is the honey-colored supernatant solution left behind when whole blood is centrifuged and the cells are separated from the plasma. While FFP can be used as a volume

expander, it carries risks of disease transmission and allergic reaction not associated with crystalloid solutions. Use FFP to treat coagulopathy related to deficiencies in clotting factors when factor-specific therapy is not available. FFP is most commonly used by emergency physicians when treating dilutional coagulopathy from severe blood loss (typically after one to two blood volumes' worth of fluid has been infused into a patient) or **DIC** (**D**isseminated **I**ntravascular **C**oagulation).

- **Platelet** preparations are used specifically for treating coagulopathy related to disorders of platelet number (thrombocytopenia) or platelet function. Like FFP, they are not typically replaced during acute blood loss unless greater than 1-2 blood volumes has already been lost. Patients may need platelets if their platelet counts are lower than 10,000-20,000 or they are showing signs of active bleeding.

Treatment – General Principles

The first and most important intervention in fluid resuscitation is the prompt administration of one or more crystalloid boluses of 20 mL/kg. During and after the administration of initial fluid boluses, assess the patient for improvement in clinical parameters, such as decrease in heart rate, improvement in distal pulses, decreased capillary refill time, or improvements in mental status. Once hemodynamically stable, consider transitioning to fluid replacement that targets maintenance, deficits, and on-going losses for correction over time.

While initial boluses are being administered, aggressively search for (and begin to treat) secondary causes of hypovolemia. For trauma patients, look for and control sources of bleeding. For patients with fever, administer *acetaminophen* or *ibuprofen* to reduce body temperature. Order laboratory studies to confirm or refute suspected diagnoses and to facilitate ongoing management.

Don't forget to monitor the volume and electrolyte status of your patients on IV therapy. A daily weight and BMP will allow you to check for volume status and to assess the adequacy of resuscitation. For patients with bleeding concerns or those receiving blood products, a CBC is mandatory, as are coagulation studies (PT/PTT) for patients receiving plasma products or at risk for coagulopathy.

Treatment – Special Considerations

Trauma

- One or more fluid boluses (20 ml/kg isotonic crystalloid)
- If still hypotensive after two fluid boluses, consider PRBC's at 10-20 mL/kg
- Extensive resuscitation (>2 blood volumes) can lead to iatrogenic coagulopathy
- Watch for oozing from previously coagulated wounds and around IV sites!
- Give FFP (10 mL/kg) and/or platelets
- Stop ongoing hemorrhage. Direct pressure, in the absence of severe coagulopathy, will stop almost all bleeding. Bandage or suture as necessary to stop the rest.

Burns

- Calculate body surface area involvement (2nd and 3rd degree burns only)
- Rough estimate: surface area of patients palm = 1% BSA
- Parkland formula
    - 24 hour requirement (mL) of *Lactated Ringer's* = 4 mL * wt (kg) * % BSA burned
    - Add maintenance fluids if <20 kg
    - Infuse first half of resuscitation fluids over 8 hours, second half over remaining 16 hours
    - Re-check electrolytes within two hours and adjust fluids as needed
- Dressing burns is important not only to prevent infection but to minimize ongoing fluid losses!

DKA

- Hyponatremia in the context of DKA is often PSEUDOHYPONATREMIA. As the *glucose* corrects, so will the *sodium*. For every 100 mg/dl *glucose* over 200, add 1.6 to the measured Na^+
- Check electrolytes and replace as necessary (e.g., *potassium*)
- Patients tend to be K^+ depleted: as acidosis corrects, serum K^+ will drop
- When blood *glucose* reaches 250 mg/dL, add *glucose*-containing fluids to prevent hypoglycemia

Fever

- Normal insensible losses are 10-30 mL/kg/day
- Insensible losses can increase 10% for each 1 degree C temperature increase

Sepsis

- Initial management of hypotension is still IV crystalloid
- Provide adequate fluids before using pressors
- Prompt antibiotic therapy is crucial to the management of sepsis from any source

Oral Rehydration

- May not be suitable for patients with continued vomiting
- Encourage small sips of a balanced electrolyte solution (such as Pedialyte)
- If patient vomits, stop fluids for one hour and then resume with small sips
- SMALL AND FREQUENT sips are the key – a 20 kg child requires 60 mL/h for maintenance fluid. This is only about four (4) tablespoons of fluid an hour (or 1 tbsp every 15 minutes)!

Hyponatremia

- Hyponatremia is common in vomiting children or infants whose lost fluids are replaced by hypotonic solutions (e.g., plain water).
- Replacement rate and fluid depend on clinical symptoms!
- For asymptomatic or mildly-symptomatic patients, correct slowly.
- For seizures due to hyponatremia more rapid correction with hypertonic *saline* is appropriate.
- Hypertonic *saline* should not be used to bring *sodium* level back to "normal" – merely to reduce clinical symptoms (risk of pontine myelinolysis).
- Calculate the *sodium* deficit (in mEq): (0.6 * weight in kg) * (140 – [serum Na])
- Correct the *sodium* at an appropriate rate based on duration of hyponatremia
    - <24 hours – rapid correction OK
    - <2 days – Max correction rate 2.5 mEq/hr
    - >2 days – Max correction rate 0.6 mEq/hr (25 mEq/48 hours)

Cardiopulmonary Disease

- Use smaller boluses – 10 mL/kg
- In these children, consider pump and rate problems as well as volume issues. Shock may not necessarily be due to (true) hypovolemia.
- Ensure adequate oxygenation

Re-assessment and Ongoing Management

- Re-assess patients frequently for response to treatment.
- For patients requiring ongoing resuscitation, consider foley catheter placement for strict monitoring of urinary output.
- If patients do not appear to be improving, re-double your search for hemorrhage, fever, GI, or other ongoing fluid losses.
- Remember to assess weights, electrolytes, and appropriate hematologic parameters on at least a daily basis.

Questions

1. Which of the following is the most important first intervention in hypovolemic shock?
   A. Stress-dose *corticosteroids*
   B. *Dopamine* at 2-10 mcg/kg/min
   C. One or more crystalloid IV fluid boluses at 20 mL/kg/min
   D. Fluid restriction
   Answer: C
2. Which of the following secondary causes of hypovolemia can be identified and treated?
   A. Sepsis
   B. Diarrhea
   C. Acute blood loss
   D. All of the above
   Answer: D
3. Why is a balanced electrolyte solution important for oral volume replacement?
   A. Rehydration with plain water alone can lead to hyponatremia and other electrolyte disturbances.
   B. Water alone causes more vomiting than balanced electrolyte solutions.

C. Balanced electrolyte solutions contain large amounts of *potassium* to counteract the effects of contraction alkalosis.

D. There is no benefit to balanced electrolyte solutions, and their use should be discouraged.

Answer: A

References

1. American College of Surgeons' Committee on Trauma, from Advanced Trauma Life Support for Doctors (ATLS) Student Manual. 2004 (7th) Edition, American College of Surgeons.
2. Carcillo JA and Tasker RC. *Fluid Resuscitation of Hypovolemic Shock: Acute Medicine's Great Triumph for Children.* Intensive Care Med (2006) 32:958-961.
3. Field JM, Hazinski MF, Gilmore D (editors). *Pediatric Advanced Life Support.* Handbook of Emergency Cardiovascular Care for Healthcare Providers (2006). American Heart Association.
4. Hillyer CD, Silberstein LE, Ness PM, Anderson KC. *Blood Banking and Transfusion Medicine: Basic Principles and Practice*, 2003. Churchill Livingstone, Philadelphia, PA.
5. Kwok, MY. Fever in the toddler. eMedicine (2006). http://www.emedicine.com/ped/topic3009.htm.
6. Marino PL and Sutin KM. *The ICU Book* (3rd edition) (2006). Lippincott Williams and Wilkins. Philadelphia, PA.
7. Preston, Richard A. *Acid-Base, Fluids, and Electrolytes Made Ridiculously Simple.* (2002). MedMaster, Inc., Miami FL.
8. Rice, H. Fluid management for the pediatric surgical patient (2006). http://www.emedicine.com/ped/topic2954.htm.

GI Surgical Emergencies

Alice Min, MD
Assistant Professor of Emergency Medicine
Department of Emergency Medicine
The University of Arizona

Malrotation/Volvulus

Critical Knowledge

Infants often present in first 3 weeks of life with bilious vomiting or signs of acute bowel obstruction. Patients may also present with signs of peritonitis or in shock. Symptoms include vomiting, which will ultimately become bilious and abdominal pain that is constant, not colicky. Patients may often have blood streaks in their stool. They may or may not have abdominal distention.

Background

- Malrotation = incomplete or abnormal rotation of the midgut during the 5th to 8th week of embryologic development
- Volvulus = twisting of midgut around the vascular stalk, causing obstruction and compromise of vascular supply
- 1 in 500 live births
- Malrotation accounts for 10% of neonatal intestinal obstruction
- Diagnosed in 75% of patients by 1 year of age

Differential Diagnoses

- Pyloric stenosis – emesis is always non-bilious; child usually appears well
- Intussusception
- Duodenal stenosis or atresia
- Incarcerated hernia
- Hirschsprung's disease

Diagnostics

- Flat and upright abdominal x-rays
  - "Double bubble" sign = gas in stomach and duodenum, otherwise airless abdomen
  - May also see distended loops of bowel overriding the liver

- If stable, upper GI series can be done
  - Failure of duodenojejunal junction to cross midline, will be seen on the right side of the spine
  - Can also see abrupt ending or corkscrew tapering appearance of contrast
  - Specificity 100%, but sensitivity only 54%
- Ultrasound
  - Studies have shown finding inversion of superior mesenteric artery and superior mesenteric vein is very indicative of malrotation and possibly volvulus
  - Other US findings suggestive of volvulus include duodenal dilatation with tapering, fixed midline bowel, whirlpool sign, and dilation of distal superior mesenteric vein

Treatment

1. Prompt surgical consultation
2. IV fluid resuscitation
3. Nasogastric tube placement if signs of obstruction
4. Labs – CBC, electrolytes, blood cultures, etc.

Questions

1. Which of the following is true regarding malrotation/volvulus?
   A. Symptoms of abdominal pain and vomiting are rare
   B. Vascular supply to the midgut is never in danger when this condition occurs
   C. A "double bubble" sign may be seen on plain films
   D. Blood in the stool is necessary to make this diagnosis
   Answer: C
2. What is one symptom that helps to differentiate malrotation/volvulus from pyloric stenosis?
   A. Abdominal pain
   B. Bilious vomiting
   C. Fever
   D. Constipation
   Answer: B

References

1. Chao HC et al. Sonographic features related to volvulus in neonatal intestinal malrotaion. *J Ultrasound Med.* 2000 June; 19(6): 371-6.
2. Hay et al. *Current Diagnosis & Treatment in Pediatrics*, 18th ed. McGraw-Hill 2007.
3. Tintinalli et al. *Emergency Medicine: A Comprehensive Study Guide.* 6th ed. McGraw-Hill 2004.
4. http://www.emedicine.com/ped/topic1200.htm
5. http://www.emedicine.com/ped/topic2415.htm

Pyloric Stenosis

Critical Knowledge

Usually presents with nonbilious projectile vomiting in 2nd or 3rd week of life. Vomiting occurs just after or near end of feeding. Emesis often becomes projectile within one week of onset. Classically, patient is a hungry infant, who feeds avidly after vomiting and has failed to gain weight or lost weight. Patients may also present with severe dehydration and constipation. Classic electrolyte abnormality is hypochloremic, hypokalemic, metabolic alkalosis. Peristaltic waves may be seen traveling left to right over the abdomen during feeding. In 60-80% of cases, the mobile hard pylorus, or "olive" may be palpated in the epigastrium.

Background

- Affects 1 in 150 males, and 1 in 750 females
- More frequent in first born males
- Also known as **I**nfantile **H**ypertrophic **P**yloric **S**tenosis (**IHPS**)
- Diffuse hypertrophy and hypoplasia of the smooth muscle causes narrowing of the antrum of the stomach that is easily obstructed
- Vomiting starts at birth in about 10% of cases

Differential Diagnoses

- GERD – vomiting is usually nonforceful, nonprojectile regurgitation
- Malrotation/volvulus

Diagnostics

- Ultrasound
  - High sensitivity (90-99%) and specificity (97-100%)
  - Hypoechoic muscle ring greater than 4 mm think with a hyperdense center
- Upper GI series if ultrasound negative
  - Retention of contrast in stomach
  - Long narrow pyloric channel with double track of barium

Treatment

- IV fluid resuscitation
- Correction of electrolyte abnormalities
- Surgical consult – pyloromyotomy is curative

Questions

1. All of the following are commonly seen in patients with pyloric stenosis EXCEPT
   A. Dehydration
   B. Projectile emesis
   C. Non-bilious vomiting
   D. Normal weight gain
   Answer: D
2. Which of the following is true regarding pyloric stenosis
   A. A palpable "olive" is always present on physical exam
   B. Hypochloremic, hypokalemic, metabolic alkalosis is common
   C. Abdominal plain films are diagnostic
   D. This condition classically presents after 6 months of age
   Answer: B

References

1. Hay et al. *Current Diagnosis & Treatment in Pediatrics*, 18th ed. McGraw-Hill 2007.
2. Tintinalli et al. *Emergency Medicine: A Comprehensive Study Guide.* 6th ed. McGraw-Hill 2004.
3. http://www.emedicine.com/emerg/topic397.htm

Intussusception

Critical Knowledge

Intussusception is the most frequent cause of intestinal obstruction in the first 2 years of life. A portion of the intestine telescopes into another segment, most commonly at the ileocolic junction. The classic patient is a thriving infant between the ages of 3 and 12 months that develops recurring paroxysms of abdominal pain. Patient will be in severe pain, often drawing up their knees. Colicky pain often lasts a few minutes at a time, 10-20 minutes apart. Vomiting and diarrhea occurs soon after onset of pain in about 90% of cases. Classic "currant jelly stools," which are bloody bowel movements with mucus, are only seen in about 50% of cases. However, guaiac positive stools are almost always present. Physical exam may reveal a palpable sausage-shaped mass over the right side of the abdomen. Patient may also present with fever, lethargy, shallow respirations, and may need a septic work up as well. Complications of intussusception include intestinal hemorrhage, incarceration, necrosis, and perforation.

Background

- Male to female ratio is 4:1
- Cause is unknown in approximately 85% of cases
  - Meckel's diverticulum, intestinal polyp, lymphoma, and complications of HSP have all been found to be lead points for intussusception
  - There may also be an association with viral illnesses, possibly related to hypertrophied lymphoid tissue

Differential Diagnoses

- Gastroenteritis – usually will have more diarrhea, ill contacts
- Meckel's diverticulum – bleeding is usually painless
- Incarcerated hernia
- Testicular or ovarian torsion
- Malrotation with volvulus
- Henoch-Schonlein Purpura may coincide with or be cause of intussusception

Diagnostics

- Enemas
  - Air contrast enema may be diagnostic and curative
  - Barium and air enemas can both be diagnostic and therapeutic

- Air enemas thought to be safer due to risk of perforation and contaminating abdominal cavity with barium
- Enema is contraindicated in patients with obvious surgical abdomen or patients suspected to have strangulated bowel, perforation, or presence of severe toxicity

- There have also been studies using ultrasound to diagnose intussusception in low-risk patients

Treatment

- Surgical consult before performing diagnostic procedures
- If reduction successful, admit for observation
- There is a 3-4% recurrence rate, usually within 24 hours, after hydrostatic or pneumatic reduction

Questions

1. Which of the following have been associated with intussusception?
   A. Meckel's diverticulum
   B. Polyp
   C. Lymphoma
   D. All of the above

   Answer: D

2. All of the following are true regarding intussusception EXCEPT
   A. The classic "currant jelly" stools are seen in a majority of cases
   B. The ileocolic junction is the most common site
   C. Barium and air enemas can both be diagnostic and therapeutic
   D. Complications include intestinal hemorrhage, incarceration, necrosis, and perforation

   Answer: A

References

1. Bhisitkul et al. Clinical application of ultrasonography in the diagnosis of intussusception. *J Pediatr.* 1992 Aug; 121(2): 182-6.
2. Hay et al. *Current Diagnosis & Treatment in Pediatrics*; 18th ed. McGraw-Hill 2007.
3. Tintinalli et al. *Emergency Medicine: A Comprehensive Study Guide.* 6th ed. McGraw-Hill 2004.
4. http://www.emedicine.com/emerg/topic397.htm

Appendicitis

Critical Knowledge

Pediatric patients often do not present with classical symptoms of abdominal pain localizing to the right lower quadrant and anorexia. Children may present with a variety of symptoms and with varied progression of symptoms, including fever, diffuse abdominal tenderness, irritability, constipation, diarrhea, vomiting, and refusal to walk. Because of these vague symptoms, the incidence of perforation at the time of presentation is high (40%). Other conditions may mimic appendicitis and physical findings may be inconclusive. Therefore, it is important to perform repeated abdominal exams over several hours. Walking, jumping up and down, and climbing onto the stretcher may all cause pain. Temperature and white blood cell count may be normal.

Background

- Most common nontraumatic pediatric surgical emergency
- More common over age of 2 years old
- Peak incidence 9-12 years of age

Differential Diagnoses

- Gastroenteritis
- UTI
- Intussusception
- PID

Diagnostics

- Ultrasound: with experienced sonographers, US has sensitivity of 85% and specificity of 94%
- CT scan: one study showed sensitivity and specificity of CT to be 94% and 95%, respectively, which was superior to US

Treatment

- Surgical consultation
- Resuscitate with IV fluids
- Labs – CBC, urinalysis, pregnancy test
- Broad spectrum antibiotics if perforation is suspected

Questions

1. Which of the following is true regarding appendicitis?
   A. Pediatric patients often present with classic symptoms of appendicitis, similar to adults
   B. Fever and elevated white blood cell counts are always present
   C. Perforation at the time of presentation is very rare
   D. Walking, jumping up and down, and climbing onto the stretcher may all cause pain

   Answer: D

2. Which of the following is appropriate in the management of appendicitis?
   A. IV fluid resuscitation
   B. Surgical consultation
   C. Urinalysis and CBC
   D. All of the above

   Answer: D

References

1. Doria AS et al. *US or CT for diagnosis of appendicitis in children and adults? A meta-analysis.* Radiology. 2006 Oct; 241(1): 83-94.
2. Hay et al. *Current Diagnosis & Treatment in Pediatrics*; 18th ed. McGraw-Hill 2007.
3. Tintinalli et al. *Emergency Medicine: A Comprehensive Study Guide.* 6th ed. McGraw-Hill 2004.
4. http://www.emedicine.com/EMERG/topic361.htm

Meckel's Diverticulum

Critical Knowledge

Most commonly presents with painless acute lower GI bleeding in children younger than 5 year of age. Intestinal obstruction is also present in 25-40% of pediatric patients. Heterotopic mucosa in diverticulum is most commonly gastric (80%), but may also be pancreatic, ileal, jejunal, or colonic. Bleeding often results from ulceration of gastric mucosa. Meckel's diverticulum may also be lead point causing intussusception. Acute inflammation of diverticulum may mimic appendicitis.

Background

- Incidence approximately 2%
- Classically presents in patients younger than 2 years
- Results from incomplete obliteration of the omphalomesenteric duct, connecting the midgut to the yolk sac
- This is a true diverticulum – contains all layers of intestinal wall

Differential Diagnoses

- Appendicitis
- Intussusception
- Malrotation with volvulus
- Anal fissure
- Bacterial enteritis

Diagnostics

- Plain abdominal x-ray
  - May show signs of obstruction or perforation
  - May be normal
- Meckel scan
  - Radionuclide imaging technique using technetium-99 m-pertechnetate which is taken up by heterotopic gastric mucosa in the diverticulum
  - Noninvasive
  - Involves less radiation exposure than that from and upper GI series and small bowel follow-through study
  - Sensitivity ranges from 75-100%
  - Specificity more than 80%
  - Meckel diverticulum must be actively bleeding at a minimum rate of 0.1 mL per minute in order to be visualized

Treatment

- Resuscitate with IV fluids
- Transfuse with blood products if needed
- Nasogastric tube placement if bowel obstruction is present
- Surgical consultation

Questions

1. Which of the following is true regarding Meckel's diverticulum?
   A. Commonly presents with painful lower GI bleeding
   B. Heterotopic mucosa in diverticulum is most commonly gastric
   C. Does not contain all layers of the intestinal wall
   D. Rarely seen as lead point in intussusception

   Answer: B
2. Which of the following is true regarding a Meckel scan?
   A. Invasive
   B. Involves more radiation than upper GI series
   C. Bleeding must be present to identify Meckel's diverticulum
   D. Radionuclide imaging technique using technetium-99 m-pertechnetate which is taken up by heterotopic pancreatic mucosa

   Answer: C

References

1. Tintinalli et al. *Emergency Medicine: A Comprehensive Study Guide.* 6th edition. McGraw-Hill 2004.
2. http://www.emedicine.com/ped/topic1389.htm

Necrotizing Enterocolitis

Critical Knowledge

Necrotizing enterocolitis primarily affects the GI tract, but may also have serious systemic effects. Typically, this condition is seen in the NICU in premature infants within the first few weeks of life. Occasionally, term infants may be affected, with the average age of onset within the first week of life. Term neonates with NEC are usually systemically ill with other predisposing conditions, such as birth asphyxia, respiratory distress, congenital heart disease, metabolic abnormalities, or a history of abnormal fetal growth pattern. Initial symptoms may be subtle and can include feeding intolerance, delayed gastric emptying, abdominal distention, ileus, decreased bowel sounds, abdominal wall erythema (late finding), and hematochezia. Systemic signs may be nonspecific and can include apnea, lethargy, decreased peripheral perfusion, shock, and cardiovascular collapse.

Background

- Most common gastrointestinal medical and/or surgical emergency occurring in neonates
- Incidence is inversely related to birth weight and gestational age
- Mortality higher in premature infants
- Cause is unknown
- No single organism has been identified as trigger
- Has also been associated with anoxic episode
- Ischemia and/or reperfusion may play a role in development of condition as well

Differential Diagnoses

- Hirschsprung disease
- Malrotation with volvulus
- Sepsis

Diagnostics

- Plain abdominal x-ray
- Pneumatosis intestinalis (air within bowel wall) is pathognomonic
- Hepatic portal air
- Intrabdominal free air if perforation has already occurred

Treatment

- IV fluid resuscitation
- Broad-spectrum antibiotics
- NPO
- Surgical consultation

Questions

1. Which of the following is true regarding necrotizing enterocolitis?
   A. Pneumatosis intestinalis is pathognomonic
   B. Most commonly affects term infants
   C. Systemic effects like shock are rarely seen
   D. Antibiotics are not indicated

   Answer: A

2. All of the following are associated with necrotizing enterocolitis EXCEPT
   A. Prematurity
   B. Anoxic episode
   C. Feeding intolerance
   D. All are associated with NEC

   Answer: D

References

1. Tintinalli et al. *Emergency Medicine: A Comprehensive Study Guide*. 6th ed. McGraw-Hill 2004.
2. http://www.emedicine.com/ped/topic2601.htm

Hirschsprung Disease

Critical Knowledge

In neonates, history often includes delayed passage of meconium (greater than 48 hours), abdominal distention, and repeated vomiting. Older children often present with symptoms of chronic constipation. Patients may be malnourished, resulting from abdominal distention, early satiety, and discomfort due to chronic constipation. Hirschsprung enterocolitis is a fatal complication of Hirschsprung disease and typically presents with abdominal pain, vomiting, fever, foul-smelling or bloody diarrhea. Enterocolitis may progress to sepsis, transmural intestinal necrosis, and perforation if not recognized early. Physical exam often reveals tympanitic abdominal distention and symptoms of intestinal obstruction. Rectal exam often reveals an empty rectal vault.

Background

- Occurs in approximately 1 in 5,000 live births
- 4 times more common in males than females
- Nearly all children with Hirschsprung disease are diagnosed by 2 years of age
- Ganglion cells are derived from the neural crest. They migrate caudally with the vagal nerve fibers along the intestine and arrive in the proximal colon by 8 weeks of gestational age and in the rectum by 12 weeks of gestational age. Failure of complete migration leads to an aganglionic segment.
- Overall mortality of Hirschsprung enterocolitis is 25-30%
- Family history of this condition may be present

- Strong association with Down's Syndrome

Differential Diagnoses

- Constipation from other cause
- Malrotation with volvulus
- Gastroenteritis
- Meconium plug syndrome

Diagnostics

- Plain abdominal x-ray, may show signs of obstruction
- Barium enema
  - May show a transition zone between a narrowed aganglionic segment and a dilated and normally innervated segment
  - May also reveal a nondistensible rectum (classic sign of Hirschsprung disease)
- Rectal biopsy provides a definitive diagnosis

Treament

- IV fluid resuscitation
- Nasogastric tube placement if suspected obstruction
- NPO
- Broad-spectrum antibiotics for patient with enterocolitis
- Surgical consultation

Questions

1. Which of the following are true regarding Hirschsprung disease?
   A. Definitive diagnosis is made by plain abdominal x-ray
   B. Results from embryologic failure to develop intestinal smooth muscle
   C. Constipation is a rare symptom
   D. History may include delayed passage of meconium

   Answer: D

2. Which diagnostic study provides a definitive diagnosis of Hirschsprung disease?
   A. Abdominal plain film
   B. Barium enema
   C. CT scan
   D. Rectal biopsy

   Answer: D

References

1. http://www.emedicine.com/ped/topic1010.htm

Blunt Abdominal Trauma

Mike Hudson, MD
Assistant Professor of Emergency Medicine
Department of Emergency Medicine
The University of Arizona

Critical Knowledge

- Have a high index of suspicion, children with no outward signs of injury may have serious intra-abdominal pathology. Half of children with blunt intestinal injury have no peritoneal signs.
- ABC's, IV, O2, monitor
- Establish IV access quickly – an intraoseous line is indicated, in the ill patient, if access can't be established after two tries or 60 seconds. Administer two 20 ml/kg boluses, repeat once more and/or give blood products if continued hypotension or tachycardia.
- Perform abdominal exam, plain films, and FAST as soon as possible and then determine the next branch point.
  - Observation and serial exams – stable patient with benign exam
  - CT scan – stable patient with questionable exam, severe mechanism, or continued high index of suspicion
  - Immediate surgical intervention – positive FAST, free air, or unstable patient.

Epidemiology/Anatomy

Anatomical differences in children make them more vulnerable to major abdominal injuries with very minor forces. In children, the abdomen begins at the level of the nipple. Children's small, pliable rib cages and undeveloped abdominal muscles provide little protection of major organs. Solid organs (e.g., spleen, liver, kidneys) are vulnerable to injury.

Differential/Critical Concepts

Abdominal Wall Bruising

Bruising of the abdominal wall after motor vehicle collision is an important finding. The sensitivity, specificity, positive predictive value, and negative predictive value for a significant intra-abdominal injury are 73.5%, 98.8%, 11.5%, and 99.9%, respectively. About 9 children with abdominal wall bruising need to be evaluated to diagnose one significant intra-abdominal injury (NNT=9).

Stomac Injuries

Blunt injuries to the stomach occur more frequently in children than in adults. The injury is usually a blowout or perforation of the greater curvature. Children who are struck by a vehicle or who fall across bicycle handlebars shortly after eating a meal are at greater risk. Consider injury to the stomach if the child has peritoneal signs and/or bloody nasogastric drainage. Abdominal x-ray films may show pneumoperitoneum.

Small Intestinal Injury

The most common intra-abdominal organ injured in restrained children involved in MVCs. Rapid deceleration may cause the lap belt to compress the intestines against the spine. An increase in intraluminal pressure may lead to rupture or tear.

- Duodenal injuries are rare, a coiled spring appearance on contrasted CT is suggestive
- Occurs in the areas of fixation at the Treitz ligament or at the ileocecal valve. Up to 50% of children with lap seat belt injuries have associated retroperitoneal injuries. Flexion-distraction lumbar spine injury may also occur.
- **Beware** – it is common for these to present as a delayed finding in children (24-48 hours post trauma)

Rectal Injuries

Except for the occasional straddle injury, child abuse or sexual activity causes most isolated rectal injuries in children.

Splenic Injuries

Splenic injuries are relatively common in pediatric trauma. After CT categorization of injury most patients with splenic injuries respond to nonoperative management.

Hepatic Injury

Most are managed non-operatively, after CT classification and surgical consultation. The exception, of course, is for children with a massive hepatic injury or with perihepatic vascular involvement who are not hemodynamically stable and transfusion requirements of greater than 25-40 mL/kg/d.

Pancreatic Injury

Blunt trauma causes most pancreatic injuries. A frequently cited mechanism involves falling into bicycle handlebars. CT scanning is a useful diagnostic modality in evaluating most pancreatic trauma. Operative exploration or ERCP may be needed to diagnose and treat ductal injury. Amylase and Lipase are neither sensitive nor specific in the diagnosis of pancreatic injury, however, a high level of either is suggestive.

Renal Injury

Blunt abdominal trauma involves renal injury in 10-20% of cases. The pediatric kidney is more susceptible to blunt injury due to the relative lack of perirenal fat and decreased protection from incompletely ossified ribs. Contusion is the most common renal injury encountered in children.

The concept of nonoperative management has been expanded to include renal injuries as well. Conservative management is standard for low-grade renal injury (grades I-III). A treatment strategy adopted by some Level I trauma centers includes bed rest for 24 hours, serial hematocrit, heart rate monitoring, and frequent physical examinations.

Management of high-grade renal injury is more controversial (grades IV-V). Absolute indications for renal exploration are an expanding or pulsatile renal hematoma. Relative indications include urinary extravasation, nonviable tissue, arterial injury, and the need for complete staging. The presence or absence of hematuria and the amount thereof do not correlate with the severity of renal injury. There are reports of successful nonoperative management of grade IV injuries. All grade V injuries required operative management and only 30% achieved long-term renal salvage.

Treatment

Solid Organ Injury Management

Nonoperative management is considered the standard of care for most children with blunt solid organ injury who are clinically stable. A recent review by Holmes et al sought to identify factors predicting failure of nonoperative management. Data was collected from a 5-year multiinstitutional review of 1,818 pediatric patients who sustained splenic, hepatic, pancreatic, or renal trauma. Overall incidence of nonoperative management failure was 5%. The reasons for declaration of failure were shock, peritonitis, persistent hemorrhage, pancreatic injury, hollow viscus injury, and ruptured diaphragm. Overall mortality for this cohort was 0.8%, with those patients in the failure group. Time to failure was 59% by 4 hours and 87% by 24 hours. A significantly increased risk of failure was associated with bicycle-related mechanism of injury, isolated pancreatic injury, and isolated grade 5 injury. Multiple solid organ injuries were associated with a higher risk of failure as well.

The data emphasize the importance of early vigilance in the care of the child with a solid organ injury. Those who will fail nonoperative management will likely do so early, within the first 12 hours. An important finding is that pancreatic injuries do not behave as other solid organs injured and are associated with a higher need for operative intervention. For isolated liver or spleen injury, current recommendations for length of stay and observation are per Stylianos and the American Pediatric Surgical Association (APSA). These recommendations are based on CT grade of injury. For grade 1 injury, no ICU stay, 2 total hospital days, and 3 weeks activity restriction. For grade 2 injury, no ICU stay, 3 total hospital days, and 4 weeks activity restriction. For grade 3 injury, no ICU stay, 4 total hospital days, and 5 weeks activity restriction. For grade 4 injury, 1 day of ICU stay, 5 total hospital days, and 6 weeks of activity restriction. These guidelines have been prospectively evaluated and demonstrate significant reduction in length of stay without adverse sequelae.

Management of Hollow Viscus Injuries

As stated earlier, these injuries are often missed on the initial assessment of children involved in blunt trauma. Have a high index of suspicion, especially if there is a significant mechanism. If there is any question after serial exams and labs, a surgical consult should be obtained.

Questions

1. Is abdominal wall bruising sensitive for intra abdominal injury in pediatric patients?

   Answer: Yes

2. What is the most frequently missed injury in children with blunt abdominal trauma?

   Answer: Hollow viscus

3. Is CT sensitive for hollow viscus injury in children?

   Answer: No

4. When should an intraosseos line be considered?

   Answer: After two peripheral attempts and/or 60 seconds

References

1. *Pediatric Duodenal Perforation Missed on Computed Tomography*, www.sciencedirect.com/#afn2. Robert Barandica, MD and Mitesh Patel, MD.
2. Splenic Injury: Trends in Evaluation and Management. *Journal of Trauma-Injury Infection & Critical Care*. 44(2):283-286, February 1998. Brasel, Karen J. MD, MPH; DeLisle, Christine M. MD; Olson, Christine J. MD; Borgstrom, David C. MD.
3. E-Medicine Abdominal Trauma, Blunt Blunt Joseph A Salomone III, MD, Jeffrey P Salomone, MD, NREMT-P
4. Imaging gastrointestinal perforation in pediatric blunt abdominal trauma. Pediatric Radiology. D. H. Jamieson, P. S. Babyn and R. Pearl.
5. Clinical recognition and management of pediatric blunt abdominal trauma without ultrasound or computed tomography scan in community hospitals in Mexico. Porras-Ramírez G, Ramírez-Reyes F, Hernández-Herrera MH, Porras-Hernández JD
6. Diagnostic and therapeutic consequences of kidney injuries in pediatric blunt abdominal trauma. Wessel LM, Jester I, Scholz S, Arnold R, Lorenz C, Wirth H, Waag KL. Acedemic Emergency Medicine. FAST Exams in Pediatric Abdominal Trauma Chris S Kennedy and Jeff Kempf.

Hematologic Emergencies

James Lehman, MD
Attending Physician
Emergency Physicians of Manhattan, LLC

Acute Anemia

Critical Knowledge

Background/Epidemiology/Anatomy

- Low **R**ed **B**lood **C**ell (**RBC**) count as assessed by hemoglobin and hematocrit
  - Must be determined using age-adjusted norms
  - Not a true disorder, but the presenting sign of many disease processes
- Incidence is 2-3 per 100 in the U.S.
- Iron deficiency anemia is by far the most common cause of anemia in children
- Age, sex, and racial predominance varies by the disease process
  - Common anemias by age
    - Newborns
      - Blood loss at birth
      - Prematurity (causes an earlier nadir in hemoglobin levels)
      - Isoimmune hemolytic disease of the newborn
      - Congenital red cell disorders
    - Infants
      - Iron deficiency anemia
      - Nutritional anemias
      - **T**ransient **E**rythroblastopenia of **C**hildhood (**TEC**)
    - Young children
      - Iron deficiency anemia
      - Infectious anemias (e.g., Parvovirus B19, Epstein-Barr Virus)
      - Autoimmune hemolytic anemias
      - TEC

        - Adolescents
            - Iron deficiency anemia
            - Nutritional anemias
            - Menstruation related anemia
    - Sex variations
        - X-linked disorders such as hemophilia and ***G****lucose*-**6**-**P**hosphate **D**ehydrogenase (**G6PD**) deficiency affect males
        - Von Willebrand's disease may cause heavy menses in females
    - Racial variations
        - Alpha-thalassemia affects Asian, Middle Eastern, and African-American populations
        - Beta-thalassemia affects Mediterranean and Middle Eastern populations
        - Sickle cell anemia affects African-American populations
        - G6PD deficiency affects African American and Mediterranean populations

Differential Diagnosis

- Inadequate RBC production
    - Bone marrow failure
        - Anemia of chronic disease
        - Aplastic anemia (e.g., Parvovirus B19 infection, idiopathic, etc.)
        - Chronic renal or liver disease
        - Drugs (e.g., chemotherapeutic agents, antiepileptics)
        - **T**ransient **E**rythroblastopenia of **C**hildhood (**TEC**)
        - Congenital red cell aplasia (e.g., Diamond-Blackfan Syndrome)
        - Malignant bone marrow infiltration (e.g., leukemia, lymphoma)
        - Hypothyroidism
        - Fanconi anemia
    - Defective hemoglobin synthesis
        - Iron deficiency anemia
        - Lead poisoning
        - Nutrient deficiencies (e.g., *pyridoxine*, copper)
    - Defective DNA synthesis

        - B_{12}/folate deficiency
        - Drugs (e.g., *phenytoin*, *trimethoprim*, *methotrexate*)
- Increased RBC destruction (hemolysis)
    - Hemolytic anemias
        - Isoimmune hemolytic disease of the newborn (i.e., Rh factor incompatibility, seen with Rh(-) mothers)
        - Autoimmune
            - Idiopathic
            - Autoimmune disease (e.g., SLE, rheumatoid arthritis)
            - Infection (e.g., Epstein-Barr Virus, mycoplasma)
            - Drugs (e.g., *penicillin*, *quinidine*)
    - Membrane defects causing early destruction
        - Hereditary spherocytosis
        - Hereditary elliptocytosis
        - **P**aroxysmal **N**octurnal **H**emoglobinuria (**PNH**)
    - Hemoglobinopathies
        - Sickle cell anemia
        - Thalassemias
    - Enzymopathies
        - G6PD deficiency
        - Pyruvate kinase dcficiency
    - Other causes
        - Microangiopathic anemia (DIC, HUS, TTP, HELLP Syndrome)
        - Mechanical destruction (e.g., artificial heart valve)
        - Hypersplenism
        - Toxins (e.g., snake bite)
        - Thermal burns
        - Infections (e.g., malaria)
- RBC loss from bleeding
- Blood loss at birth (e.g., birth trauma, twin-twin transfusion, maternal-fetal transfusion)
- GI bleeding
- Menstrual bleeding

- Traumatic blood loss
- Coagulation defects (e.g., hemophilia, Von Willebrand's disease)

Critical Concepts

- Age is an important factor when diagnosing anemia in children
  - Hemoglobin levels peak at birth and hit a nadir within 2-3 months
  - Nadir occurs earlier in premature infants
  - Diagnosis of "anemia" must be made using age-adjusted norms
  - Age determines the most likely causes of anemia (see above)
- History can be a key to diagnosis
  - Birth history—prematurity, blood loss at birth, twinning, excessive bleeding at circumcision or from umbilical cord (hemophilia)
  - Family history—anemias, splenectomy, inherited disorders, need for transfusions
  - Ethnicity and race (see previous)
  - Diet/feeding history
    - Infants
      - Iron-fortified vs. non-fortified formula
      - Breast-feeding—normally adequate for 6 months
      - Whole milk—not a good source of iron, may cause GI bleeding
    - Older children
      - Sources of iron: meats, cereal, green vegetables
      - Excessive soda and fatty snacks have been associated with anemia
      - Assess for eating disorders
  - Growth history—poor growth may signal anemia of chronic disease
  - Medications (e.g., chemotherapeutic agents, antiepileptics, *pencicillin*, trimethaprim, etc.)
  - Pica—eating inedible substances such as dirt or paint chips, may signify iron deficiency
  - Lead based paints at home

- Clinical signs/symptoms
  - Anemia
    - Symptoms—pallor, weakness, malaise, lethargy, lightheadedness, anorexia
    - Signs—tachycardia, tachypnea, systolic ejection murmur
    - In severe anemia CHF may occur with cardiomegaly, hepatomegaly, hypotension and auscultative gallop
  - Jaundice, dark urine→ hemolysis
  - Petechiae, purpura→ hemophilia, microangiopathic diseases, autoimmune hemolysis
  - Splenomegaly→ malignant infiltration, hemolysis, Epstein-Barr Virus
  - Dysmorphic face and/or limbs→ congenital diseases (e.g., Diamond-Blackfan Syndrome, Fanconi anemia)
  - Frontal bone prominence ("bossing")→ chronic hemolysis with extramedullary hematopoiesis (esp. thalassemia)
  - Hypothermia, thin hair, dry skin, failure to thrive→ hypothyroidism
  - Glossitis→B_{12} deficiency and iron deficiency
  - Diagnostic findings
    - CBC findings
      - Anemia—based on age-adjusted norms
      - Pancytopenia→aplastic anemia, microangiopathic anemia, chemotherapeutic agents
      - Pancytopenia except elevated/normal lymphcytes→leukemia
    - **M**ean **C**orpuscular **V**olume (**MCV**)
      - Elevated MCV (macrocytic anemia)→ B12/folate deficiency, hypothyroidism, reactive reticulocytosis (from RBC loss)
      - Decreased MCV (microcytic anemia)→iron deficiency, anemia of chronic disease, thalassemia
    - Corrected reticulocyte count
      - Corrected retic: count = (patient Hgb/normal Hgb) X (retic %)
      - Elevated—signifies increased RBC production by marrow in response to a loss of red cells→hemolysis, acute blood loss
      - Decreased—signifies inadequate RBC production by the marrow→marrow failure anemias (see above)

- Peripheral smear
  - Schistocytes→microangiopathic anemia
  - Ghost/bite cells→G6PD deficiency
  - Target cells (leptocytes)→hemoglobinopathies, thalassemias
  - Elliptocytes→hereditary elliptocytosis
  - Spherocytes→hereditary spherocytosis, autoimmune hemolytic anemias
  - Basophilic stippling→lead poisoning, reticulocytosis
  - Sickled cells→sickle-cell anemia
  - Heinz bodies→hemolytic anemias
  - Blast cells→malignant bone marrow infiltration
- Further testing is directed by age, clinic findings and above tests
  - LDH, bilirubin→hemolysis
  - Iron, ferritin, and total iron binding→iron deficiency anemia
  - Direct/indirect Coombs test→autoimmune hemolytic anemia
  - Hemoglobin electrophoresis→hemoglobinopathies, thalassemias
  - RBC enzyme studies→enzymopathies
  - B12 and folate levels→ B12/folate deficiency
  - Osmotic fragility testing→spherocytosis
  - Blood typing with crossmatch→isoimmune hemolytic disease of the newborn
  - Bone marrow biopsy→malignant bone marrow infiltration
  - TSH/free T4→hypothyroidism
  - Stool occult→GI bleeding
- Imaging—rarely useful in initial screening for anemia

Treatment

- Should be directed at the cause of anemia
- Supportive care
  - **P**acked **R**ed **B**lood **C**ell (**PRBC**) transfusions (10-15 ml/kg) as necessary
  - Stop medications which may cause anemia

- Iron deficiency anemia
  - Diagnosis is often made presumptively in otherwise healthy children with microcytic anemia and otherwise normal CBC and peripheral smear findings
  - Iron supplementation: 3-6 mg of elemental Iron /kg/d
  - If RBC count and MCV are not improving at 1 month follow-up, other diagnoses should be considered
- Anemia from marrow failure (e.g., chronic disease, renal disease, chemotherapeutic agents)
  - *Erythropoietin* 50-250 units/kg SC/IV 1-3 times weekly
  - Not indicated for acute anemia as effects take 2-8 weeks

Questions

1. Which is not associated with autoimmune hemolytic anemia?
   A. Positive Coombs testing
   B. Elevated corrected reticulocyte count
   C. Blast cells on peripheral smear
   D. Elevated LDH
   Answer: C
2. Which supports the diagnosis of iron deficiency anemia?
   A. Child only 1 month old, formula fed
   B. Macrocytosis on peripheral smear
   C. Jaundice and splenomegaly are noted on exam
   D. Anemia improved after one month of ferrous sulfate treatment
   Answer: D

References

1. Adams WG, Geva J, Coffman J, Palfrey S, Bauchner H. Anemia and Elevated Lead Levels in Under-immunized Inner-city Children. *Pediatrics.* 1998 Mar; 101(3):E6
2. Alexander SR. Pediatric Uses of Recombinant human Erythropoietin: the Outlook in 1991. *Am J Kidney Dis.* 1991 Oct; 18(4):42-53
3. Boutry M, Needlman R. Use of Dietary History in the Screening of Iron Deficiency. *Pediatrics.* 1996 Dec; 6(1):1138-42

Acute Leukemia

Critical Knowledge

Background/Epidemiology/Anatomy

- A malignancy resulting from clonal proliferation of a single cell line within the bone marrow
- The most common childhood malignancy
- Incidence is 30-40 per 1 million in the U.S.
- Male predominance, more common in Caucasians
- Peak incidence between ages 3 and 7
- Causes remain largely unknown, but associations are
  - Genetic disease (e.g., trisomy 21, ataxia telangiectasia, etc.)
  - Environmental factors (e.g., ionizing radiation, benzene, chemotherapeutic agents)

Differential Diagnosis

- Aplastic anemia
- Idiopathic thrombocytopenia purpura
- Juvenile rheumatoid arthritis
- Infectious mononucleosis
- Infectious leukocytosis
- Disseminated intravascular coagulation
- Malignancies
  - **A**cute **M**yelocytic **L**eukemia (**AML**)
  - Non-Hodgkin's lymphoma
  - Neuroblastoma
  - Rhabdomyosarcoma

Critical Concepts

- Leukemia is a progressive cancer that proliferates at the expense of other bone marrow cell lines (i.e., neutrophils, thrombocytes, erythrocytes)
  - Signs/symptoms of disease are a result of this lymphocytosis, with resulting neutropenia, thrombocytopenia, and anemia
- Clinical signs/symptoms—often insidious
  - General—fatigue, malaise, weight loss, low-grade fever, bone pain

- Pulmonary—dyspnea
- Hematologic—pallor, petechiae, easy bruising, mucosal bleeding, lymphadenopathy
- Renal—oliguria, occasional testicular pain/enlargement (from infiltration)
- Gastroentestinal—splenomegaly
- CNS—headache, vomiting, lethargy, nuchal rigidity, seizures, papilledema (found in CNS involvement—not common at time of initial diagnosis)

- Diagnostic findings
  - Leukocytosis—present at diagnosis in only 50% of cases
  - Neutropenia, thrombocytopenia, anemia
  - Peripheral smear—shows lymphoblasts and other immature forms
    - This is diagnostic (although bone marrow aspirate is used to confirm diagnosis)
    - Should be examined by a trained hematologist
  - Coagulation studies—generally normal
  - Electrolyte abnormalities—hyperuricemia, hyperphosphatemia, hyperkalemia, hypocalemia/hypercalemia
  - Elevated liver function tests with leukemic infiltration
  - Elevated lactate dehydrogenase (may indicate pending tumor lysis syndrome)
  - Cerebrospinal fluid—for evidence of CNS infiltration
  - CXR—may show a mediastinal mass in a 5-10% of patients
  - Bone marrow aspirate—for ultimate diagnosis, staging, and molecular analysis
- High-risk features—worse long-term prognosis
  - Age <1 year or >10 years
  - WBC count >50,000 mm3 at diagnosis
  - Male sex (testicular disease likely the reason)
  - Black race
  - Large lymphadenopathy or splenomegaly at diagnosis
  - Certain chromosomal abnormalities and antigenic expression patterns

Treatment

- Supportive care
  - Hydration therapy without *potassium* replacement
  - Blood transfusions as necessary
- Infection
  - Use broad coverage antibiotics for identified infection
  - Neutropenia requires *trimethoprim*/sulfamethoxazole prophylaxis for Pneumocystis jiroveci (PCP)
  - Neutropenia with fever requires antibiotics, admission, and isolation
- Chemotherapy induction therapy (initiated by a pediatric oncologist)
  - Three or four drug regimen determined by phenotypical findings and risk stratification.
  - Intrathecal *methotrexate* added for CNS treatment or prophylaxis
  - Can achieve remission rates >90%
- Bone marrow transplant—a treatment option for relapse
- **T**umor **L**ysis **S**yndrome (**TLS**)—a triad a hyperuricemia, hyperkalemia, and hyperphosphatemia
  - Caused by rapid cellular destruction with resulting release of large quantities of *potassium*, phosphate and urea (may be seen before or after initiation of chemotherapy)
  - Secondary effects
    - Hypocalcemia due to down regulation
    - **A**cute **R**enal **F**ailure (**ARF**)
  - Prophylaxis
    - Maintenance fluids at twice normal rate
    - NO *potassium* supplementation in IV fluids
    - Alkalization of urine with IV *sodium bicarbonate*
  - Promotes the solubility of urea and increases its excretion
  - Goal is a urine pH of 7.0-8.0
  - Suppress uric acid formation
    - *Allopurinol* 50-100 mg PO Q8 hrs
    - Recombinant urate oxidase (*rasburicase*: 0.15-0.2 mg/kg/day IV over 30 minutes)

- Monitor EKG for hyperkalemic changes (e.g., peaked T-waves, widened QRS)
- Treatment
  - Hyperkalemia
    - *Calcium gluconate* 10% (0.5 ml/kg IV over 2-5 minutes) if EKG changes are seen
    - *Sodium bicarbonate* (1-2 mEq/kg IV over 5-10 minutes)
    - *Insulin/glucose* (0.1 unit/kg IV regular *insulin* with 2 ml/kg IV D25
    - *Sodium polystyrene resin* (i.e., *kayexalate*) (1-2 g/kg with *sorbitol* PO)
    - *Furosemide* (0.5-2 mg/kg IV bolus)
    - Dialysis
  - Hyperphosphatemia
    - *Aluminum hydroxide* (50-150 mg/kg/day PO divided every 4-6 hours)
    - *Mannitol* 0.25-1 g/kg IV bolus in normal *saline*
    - Dialysis
  - Hyperuricemia
    - *Allopurinol* (10 mg/kg/d PO/IV in 3-4 divided doses) decreases urea production
    - Recombinant urate oxidase: *Rasburicase*: 0.15-0.2 mg/kg/day IV infusion over 30 minutes) increases urea excretion by converting it to allantoin, a compound with 5 times the solubility of urea
    - Alkalization of urine
- Survival rate with treatment is 80%
  - Prognosis depends heavily on genetic factors
  - Overall highest survival rates are seen in children ages 1-10

Questions

1. Which is an uncommon finding in patients with newly diagnosed ALL?
   A. Hyperkalemia
   B. Hypocalcemia
   C. Hypophosphatemia
   D. Hyperuricemia
   Answer: C

2. Which is considered a low-risk feature of ALL?
   A. Age 4 at diagnosis
   B. Male sex
   C. WBC count of 62,000 mm^3 at diagnosis
   D. 3 cm lymph nodes at diagnosis

   Answer: A

References

1. Goldman SC, Holcenberg JS, Finklestein JZ, Hutchinson R, Kreissman S, Johnson FL, Tou C, Harvey E, Morris E, Cairo MS. *A Randomized Comparison Between Rasburicase and Allopurinol in Children With Lymphoma or Leukemia at High Risk for Tumor Lysis*. Blood. 2001 May; 97(10):2998-3003
2. Ries LA, Kosary CL, Hankey BF, et al. *SEER Cancer Statistics Review*, 1973-1996. Bethesda, Md: National Cancer Institute (http://seer.cancer.gov/csr/1973_1996/)
3. Pui CH, Relling MV, Downing JR. Acute Lymphoblastic Leukemia. *N Engl J Med*. 2004; 350 (15):1535-48.

Aplastic Anemia

Critical Knowledge

Consider histocompatibility testing of patient and siblings prior to non-emergent transfusions (transfusions may later impact the success of **B**one **M**arrow **T**ransplant (**BMT**)

Background/Epidemiology/Anatomy

- A condition with various causes characterized by pancytopenia (thrombocytopenia, anemia, and neutropenia) AND hypocellular bone marrow
- Incidence is 2-6 per one million in the U.S.
- No age, sex, or racial predominance
- 50% or more are idiopathic, other causes include
  A. Genetic (e.g., Fanconi anemia, Diamond-Blackfan Syndrome, etc.)
  B. Acquired
     - Infection (e.g., Epstein-Barr Virus, Parvovirus B19, HIV, hepatitis)

- Drugs (e.g., *chloramphenicol*, *sulfonamides*, *carbamazepine*, *cimetadine*, phenylbutazone, etc.)
- Toxins (e.g., radiation, benzene)
- **G**raft-**V**ersus-**H**ost **D**isease (**GVHD**)
- Others
  - Pregnancy
  - Autoimmune disease (e.g., SLE)

Differential Diagnosis

- Bone marrow infiltration (e.g., leukemia, lymphoma, myelofibrosis)
- Myelodysplasia
- Megaloblastic anemia
- Chemotherapy effects
- **P**aroxysmal **N**octurnal **H**emoglobinuria (**PND**)
- Splenic sequestration

Critical Concepts

- Pathophysiology varies and is unknown much of the time, often involves immune suppression
- Insidious onset with signs of thrombocytopenia often first noted
- Historical points
  - Family history of anemia
    - Identifying an inherited aplastic anemia can have consequences for later treatment
    - Penetrance varies making family history-taking unreliable
  - Recent infection (e.g., parvovirus, etc.)
  - Recent radiation or medication usage
- Clinical signs/symptoms
  - General—fever, weakness, lethargy, pallor
  - Hematologic—bruising, petechiae, jaundice, mucous membrane breeding
  - Gastrointestinal—GI bleeding, normal sized liver and spleen
  - Eyes—retinal hemorrhages
  - CNS—uncommon symptomatic CNS bleeding
  - Cardiovascular—systolic flow murmur

    - Developmental—abnormal facies and/or extremities seen in some congenital diseases (e.g., Fanconi anemia, Diamond-Blackfan anemia)
- Diagnostic findings
    - Anemia—macrocytic, reticulocyte count <0.1%
    - Thrombocytopenia—5,000-50,000 per ml
    - Neutropenia—with toxic granulation, no blast cells
    - Bone marrow aspirate/biopsy—hypocellular marrow
    - Folate and B12 testing
    - Specialized testing
        - Ham test— (tests stability of red cell for Paroxysmal Nocturnal Hemoglobinuria)
        - Serologic viral testing (HIV, EBV, hepatitis, etc.)
        - Autoimmune panel (e.g., SLE)
        - Chromosomal studies to rule out genetic disease

Treatment

- Supportive therapy
    - Stop exposure to all possible causative agents!
    - Blood transfusions
        - Minimize when possible—better bone marrow transplant results occur with lower rates of transfusion
        - Leuko-reduced blood products minimize alloimmunization
    - Infection treatment
        - Use broad coverage antibiotics for identified infection
        - Neutropenia requires *trimethoprim/sulfamethoxazole* prophylaxis for Pneumocystis jiroveci (PCP)
        - Neutropenia with fever requires antibiotics, admission, and isolation
- HLA-matched **B**one **M**arrow **T**ransplant (**BMT**)—therapy of choice for children with severe aplastic anemia
    - Requires an HLA-compatible sibling
    - Survival rates better than with immunosuppression therapy alone
    - Unrelated-donor BMT not nearly as successful
- Immunosuppression—when no HLA-compatible sibling is present
    - **A**nti**T**hymocyte **G**lobulin (**ATG**), high-dose *prednisone*, and *cyclosporine*

    - Combination therapy has shown better results than monotherapy
- Survival rate between 85-95% with BMT

Questions

1. Which is not a known cause of aplastic anemia?
    A. Chloramphenical
    B. Hepatitis
    C. Fanconi's anemia
    D. Folate deficiency
    Answer: D
2. Which is not a concept of aplastic anemia treatment?
    A. Broad-spectrum antibiotics for infection
    B. Blood transfusions early and often
    C. HLA-compatibility testing for patient and siblings
    D. Leuko-reduced blood products
    Answer: F

References

1. Giampietro PF, Davis JG, Adler-Brecher B, Verlander PC, Auerbach AD, Pavlakis SG. The Need for More Accurate and Timely Diagnosis in Fanconi Anemia: A Report from the International Fanconi Anemia Registry. *Pediatrics*. 1993 June; 91(6):1116-1120
2. Guinan EC. *Aplastic Anemia: The Management of Pediatric Patients.* Hematology: Am Soc Hematol Educ Program Book. 2005:104-109
3. Killick SB, Marsh JC, Gordon-Smith EC, Sorlin L, Gibson FM. *Long-term Outcome of Acquired Aplastic Anemia in Children: Comparison between Immunosuppressive Therapy and Bone Marrow Transplantation.* Br J Haematol. 2000; 111:321–328.
4. Killick SB, Win N, Marsh JC, et al. *Pilot study of HLA Alloimmunization after Transfusion with Pre-storage Leucodepleted Blood products in Aplastic Anaemia.* Br J Haematol. 1997; 97:677–684.
5. Marsh J, Schrezenmeier H, Marin P, et al. Prospective Randomized Multicenter Study Comparing Cyclosporin Alone Versus the Combination of Antithymocyte Globulin and Cyclosporin for Treatment of Patients with Nonsevere Aplastic Anemia: A Report from the European Blood and Marrow Transplant (EBMT) Severe Aplastic Anaemia Working Party. Blood. 1999; 93:2191–2195

Hemolytic Uremic Syndrome (HUS)

Critical Knowledge

- Transfuse platelets and PRBC's only when bleeding is ongoing and life threatening or if needed prior to invasive procedures
- If cardiac arrest occurs, consider hyperkalemia as a cause

Background/Epidemiology/Anatomy

- A group of diseases entities with the common triad of microangiopathic hemolytic anemia, thrombocytopenia, and acute renal failure
- Most common cause of pediatric acute renal failure
- Rare disorder with less than 1,000 new cases per year
- Peak age is under age 10, with a majority being under age 4
- Can be epidemic with clusters occurring during the summer
- No sex predominance, rare in African Americans
- Two diagnostic types with different natural histories
    - Typical (D+) HUS often occurs after a prodromal gastroenteritic illness with Shiga-toxin producing Escherichia coli (i.e., E. coli 0157:H7)
    - Atypical (D-) HUS encompasses all other forms of HUS, the pathogenesis of these is not well understood

Differential Diagnosis

- **T**hrombotic **T**hrombocytopenic **P**urpura (**TTP**)
- **D**isseminated **I**ntravascular **T**hrombosis (**DIC**)
- Hemolytic anemias with accompanying thrombocytopenia
- Vasculitis

Critical Concepts

- Clinical effects of D+ HUS are a direct result of damaged endothelial cells caused by bacterial toxins
    - Endothelial cell-wall damage leads to red blood cell hemolysis and the release of vasoactive substances
    - Thrombocytopenia results from platelet destruction and consumption at the sites of endothelial damage
    - Renal failure results from a decreased glomerular filtration rate secondary to microthrombi in the renal vasculature

- Conflicting evidence suggests antibiotic treatment of gastroenteritis caused by E. coli 0157:H7 may trigger HUS
- Clinical signs/symptoms
    - General—fever, elevated blood pressure, signs of dehydration
    - Hematologic—pallor, petechiae, purpura
    - Gastrointestinal—prodromal diarrhea (often bloody), abdominal pain, pancreatitis (usually mild)
    - Renal—decreased urine output
    - CNS—lethargy, irritability, ataxia, seizures, coma (caused by microthrombi and cerebral edema)
    - Cardiovascular—signs of heart failure, peripheral edema
- Diagnostic findings
    - Anemia—with signs of hemolysis (elevated lactate dehydrogenase and bilirubin, schistocytes, decreased haptoglobin)
    - Coagulation defects—increased fibrin split products, increased or normal fibrinogen, normal INR/PT/PTT
    - Leukocytosis—commonly found
    - Renal failure—elevated BUN and creatinine, hyponatremia, hyperkalemia, hyperphosphatemia, microscopic hematuria and proteinuria, RBC casts
    - Pancreatitis—elevated lipase and amylase
    - Microbiology—positive stool culture for E. coli 0157:H7, this has a low sensitivity
- HUS is a spectrum of disease which can range from subclinical to life-threatening, with a mortality rate of 3-12%

Treatment

- Renal care
    - Fluid volume resuscitation with strict attention to input and output
        - If hypovolemic, give normal *saline* or *lactated ringers* (patient is likely to be hyponatremic)
        - If hypervolemic, fluid restriction may be needed
    - Hyperkalemia may require treatment with *calcium gluconate, sodium bicarbonate, insulin/glucose*, and/or *kayexalate*
    - Antihypertensives can be required

- Dialysis is often needed at (peritoneal or hemodialysis)

- Transfusion
  - PRBC transfusion—for hemoglobin below 6.0-7.0 or with signs of cardiac dysfunction
  - Platelet transfusion—only for children with life-threatening bleeding or prior to invasive procedures (transfusing platelets inappropriately can worsen intravascular coagulation)
- Immunoglobulin G (2 g/kg IV over 2-5 days) has shown conflicting results and should only be given in concert with pediatric consultation
- Survival rate is 85-95% with D+ HUS, but lower with D- HUS which can often be chronic

Questions

1. Which of these is not part of the triad of HUS?
   A. Hemolysis
   B. Thrombocytopenia
   C. CNS dysfunction
   D. Acute renal failure
   Answer: C
2. Which lab finding might you expect to find with HUS?
   A. Leukocytosis
   B. Elevated conjugated bilirubin
   C. Hypernatremia
   D. Hypophosphatemia
   Answer: A

References

1. Constantinescu AR, Bitzan M, Weiss LS, Christen E, Kaplan BS, Cnaan A, Trachtman H. Non-enteropathic Hemolytic Uremic Syndrome: Causes and Short-term Course. *Am J Kidney Dis.* 2004 Jun; 43(6):976-982
2. Safdar N, Said A, Gangnon RE, Maki DG. Risk of Hemolytic Uremic Syndrome after Antibiotic Treatment of Escherichia coli 0157:H7 Enteritis: A Meta-analysis. *JAMA.* 2002 Aug; 288(8):996-1001.
3. Wong CS, Jelacic S, Habeeb RL, Watkins SL, Tarr PI. The Risk of the Hemolytic-Uremic Syndrome after Antibiotic Treatment of Escherichia coli 0157:H7 Infections. *N Engl J Med.* 2000 Jun; 342(26):1930-1936.

Hemophilia A and B

Critical Knowledge

- Do not delay factor replacement for imaging in children suspected of intracranial hemorrhage
- Bleeding around the airway requires early airway stabilization, surgical airway is relatively contraindicated

Background/Epidemiology/Anatomy

- Sex-linked, heritable bleeding disorders characterized absence or dysfunction of Factor VIII (hemophilia A) or Factor IX (hemophilia B) of the clotting cascade
- Incidence 200 per 1 million in the U.S. (80% of which are hemophilia A)
- X-linked disorders affecting males only
    - Females are generally asymptomatic carriers
    - Show X-linked inheritance although spontaneous mutations occur
- Congenital diseases with diagnosis generally in infancy or before birth
- No racial predominance

Differential Diagnosis

- **V**on **W**illebrand **D**isease (**VWD**)
- Other Factor deficiencies (Factor XI being the most common)
- Acquired Factor VIII or IX deficiencies due to inhibitor (rare)
- Vitamin K deficiency
- Child abuse
- Isolated prolonged coagulation times without bleeding
    - *Heparin* therapy
    - Factor XII deficiency

Critical Concepts

- Factors VIII and IX are necessary for clot formation
    - Both are involved in the intrinsic pathway of the clotting cascade
    - Absence of or abnormal function of either causes abnormal bleeding
- Severity of disease is based on the severity of factor deficiency
    - Mild—factor activity 5-25% (of normal)
    - Moderate—factor activity 1-5%

- Severe—factor activity <1%
- Clinical signs/symptoms—vary with age
  - Neonates
    - Bleeding from umbilical site or after circumcision is often the presenting sign
    - Intracranial bleeding affects 1-2% of neonates
  - Infants
    - Major bleeding is relatively uncommon
    - Mucosal bleeding, especially the lips and tongue
  - Toddlers and children
    - Hemarthrosis and soft tissue bleeding become more common
- Specific bleeding events
  - Hemarthrosis—common in weight-bearing joints (i.e., knees, ankles, elbows)
    - May start with only slight discomfort
    - Warmth, swelling, pain, and ROM limitation follow
    - Can lead to chronic arthropathy and joint destruction
  - Soft tissue bleeding—occurs at sites of minor trauma
    - Painful and may be swollen
    - Ecchymosis not always present, petechiae uncommon
    - Retroperitoneal bleeding may mimic an acute abdomen
    - Compartment syndrome may occur
  - Intracranial bleeding—even after relatively minor trauma
  - Hematuria—common and generally benign, may be persistent
  - GI bleeding—uncommon
  - Post-surgical/dental bleeding—can be life-threatening, requires prior treatment and surgeons familiar with care of hemophiliacs
- Diagnostic studies
  - Prolonged **P**artial **T**hromboplastin **T**ime (**PTT**)
    - May be normal in mild disease
    - Also prolonged in VWD
  - Normal **P**rothrombin **T**ime (**PT**), bleeding times, and platelet count

- Special testing
  - Factor VIII:C assay—low in hemophilia A
  - Factor IX assay—low in hemophilia B
  - Von Willebrand antigen assay (VWF:Ag)—normal in hemophilia, may be low in VWD

Treatment

- General concepts for acute treatment
  - Treatment of acute bleeding events is intravenous replacement of the appropriate factor
    - Factor VIII
      - 1 unit (U) of Factor VIII raises circulating levels by 2%
      - Serum half-life is 8-12 hours
    - Factor IX
      - 1 unit (U) of Factor IX raises circulating levels by 1%
      - Serum half-life is 24 hours
  - Dosing of factor replacement varies with the site and severity of injury
- Factor replacement
  - Recombinant factors
    - Now standard treatment for newly diagnosed patients
    - Low or no risk of blood borne pathogens (e.g., HIV, hepatitis)
  - Concentrated plasma-derived factors
    - Slightly higher risk of blood borne pathogens
    - Cheaper than newer recombinant treatments
    - Not recommended for newly diagnosed patients or those who have been previously maintained on recombinant factors
- Factor replacement therapy for specific injuries
  - Hemarthosis—level of activity required is 30-50%
    - Factor VIII 20-40 U/kg
    - Factor IX 30-40 U/kg
    - Other: consider immobilization, orthopedic consultation
  - Muscular bleeding—level of activity required is 40-50%
    - Factor VIII 20-40 U/kg
    - Factor IX 40-60 U/kg

        - Other: elevate area, observe for compartment syndrome
    - Epistaxis—level of activity required is 80-100%
        - Factor VIII 40-50 U/kg
        - Factor IX 80-100 U/kg
        - Other: treat bleeding appropriately
    - Oral bleeding— level of activity required is 50%
        - Factor VIII 25 U/kg
        - Factor IX 50 U/kg
        - Other: aminocaproic acid
    - GI bleeding— level of activity required is 100%
        - Factor VIII 40-50 U/kg
        - Factor IX 80-100 U/kg
        - Other: consult gastroenterology
    - Intracranial bleeding—level of activity required is 100%
        - Factor VIII 50 U/kg
        - Factor IX 100 U/kg
        - Other: consult neurosurgery
- Inhibitors—IgG antibodies to factors VIII or IX which shorten the half-life of replacement factor
    - Inhibitors complicate the treatment of hemophilia by decreasing the effectiveness of common factor replacement therapies
    - Frequency
        - Factor VIII inhibitor occurs in up to 35% of children with severe hemophilia A
        - Factor IX inhibitor occurs only in 1-3% of children with hemophilia B
    - Inhibitors are described based on the intravenous titer levels
        - Low-level titers—can generally be treated with normal or high-dose factor replacement therapies
        - High-level titers—require alternative therapies
            - Immune tolerance induction
            - Porcine factor VIII (e.g., Hyate;C)
            - Anti-inhibitor coagulant complex (e.g., FEIBA)
            - Recombinant factor VIIa (e.g., NovoSeven)

- Other medical therapies
    - Aminocaproic acid (100 mg/kg orally every 4- 6 hours)
        - Inhibits activation of plasminogen, stabilizing clot formation
        - Useful in oral bleeding, counteracts fibrinolysin found in saliva
    - *Desmopressin* (0.3 micrograms/kg IV every 12-24 hours)
        - Dose-dependent increase in Factor VIII release
        - Effective treatment for mild to moderate hemophilia A only. Can be used for minor bleeding or prior to surgery
- Chronic (prophylactic) therapy
    - Now considered primary treatment for many patients, prophylactic factor replacement, often 3 times weekly is given to keep factor activity levels above 25%
    - This treatment may be more cost beneficial than symptomatic treatment due to decreased episodes of acute bleeding
    - This often requires IV port placement due to frequent IV administrations of factor

Questions

1. Which is not generally seen in hemophilia?
    A. Petechiae
    B. Easy bruising
    C. Oral bleeding
    D. Epistaxis

    Answer: A
2. This is the correct factor replacement dosing for a hemophilia A patient with epistaxis?
    A. 50 U/kg to replace 50% of factor activity
    B. 25 U/kg to replace 50% of factor activity
    C. 50 U/kg to replace 100% of factor activity
    D. 25 U/kg to replace 25% of factor activity

    Answer: C

References

1. Kelly KM, Butler RB, Farace L, Cohen AR, Manno CS. Superior in vivo Response of Recombinant Factor VIII Concentrate in Children with Hemophilia A. *J Pediatr.* 1997 Apr; 130(4):537-40
2. Ljung RC. *Prophylactic Infusion Regimens in the Management of Hemophilia.* Thromb Haemost. 1999 Aug; 82(2):525-30
3. Ludlam CA. *The Evidence Behind Inhibitor Treatment with Recombinant Factor VIIa.* Pathophysiol Haemost Thromb. 2002; 32 Suppl 1:13-8

Henoch-Schonlein Purpura (HSP)

Background/Epidemiology/Anatomy

- A small-vessel vasculitis causing purpura, arthralgias, and abdominal pain in children
- Incidence is 150 per 1 million in the U.S.
- Males predominance is 2:1
- Prevalence peaks between ages 4 and 15
- Peak incidence is in the spring
- Caucasians are effected more often than African-Americans

Differential Diagnosis

- Thrombocytopenia purpura (e.g., TTP, ITP)
- Meningococcemia
- Rocky Mountain Spotted Fever
- Other small vessel vasculitities (e.g., leukocytoclastic vasculitis, polyarteritis nodosa, SLE, etc.)
- Child abuse

Critical Concepts

- HSP is an Immunoglobulin A (IgA) mediated vasculitis
  - Antigens may play a role, stimulating an autoimmune response
  - Viral/bacterial antigens are suspected as children often have preceding symptoms 1-3 weeks prior to onset of HSP
- The hallmark of the disease is palpable purpura on dependent parts of the body, especially the legs and buttocks but not all patients will have this rash early on.

- Though there is no treatment for HSP a majority of children recover spontaneously over weeks months
- Clinical signs/symptoms
    - General—low-grade fever, preceding URI symptoms common
    - Hematologic—symmetrical erythematous rash in lower extremities which spreads and later becomes palpable purpura
    - Gastroentestinal (30-50% of patients)
        - GI bleeding (occasionally massive) with melena, hematochezia and/or hematemesis
        - Abdominal complaints including nausea, vomiting, diarrhea and pain (obstruction, infarction, and intussusception of the bowel can rarely occur)
    - Renal—rare oliguria or gross hematuria, scrotal/testicular pain
    - Rheumatologic (60-80% of patients)—arthralgias and arthritis, especially in the knees and ankles
    - Skin—subcutaneous edema of scalp common in infants
- Diagnostic findings
    - Diagnosis is generally clinical, but in subtle or early cases workup may be required, renal testing is mandatory if HSP is considered
    - CBC is nonspecific but may show leukocytosis, thrombocytosis, and eosinophilia
    - Renal findings can vary and occur in approx. 50% of patients
        - Glomerulonephritis—elevated creatinine, hematuria, proteinuria, RBC casts
        - Nephrotic syndrome—significant proteinuria with edema
        - Oliguria and hypertension are rare
    - Stool guiac positive in patients with GI symptoms
    - IgA levels elevated
    - Joint examinations
        - Plain films may show joint effusion
        - Effusion is serous, not bloody, if arthrocentesis is performed
    - Other imaging
        - Abdominal radiographs—bowel edema, thumbprinting
        - Ultrasound—bowel edema, free fluid, intussusception

Treatment

- Supportive care
  - Limitation of strenuous physical activity
  - Pain management
- Renal care
  - Fluid hydration
  - Low-salt diet
  - Atihypertensives
- *Azithioprine* has been used in cases of severe renal disease
  - Limited data suggests improvement in long-term renal outcome
  - Therapy generally continued for several weeks
- *Corticosteroid* therapy is not recommended unless severe renal disease occurs
  - Improves arthritic and abdominal symptoms
  - Limited data suggests improvement in long-term renal outcome
  - Increases the rate of relapse
- Survival rate is excellent at >98%
  - Chronic renal disease develops in <5% (<1% with ESRD)
  - Relapse rate is up to 50%
    - Usually occurring within 1-2 months
    - Increased rate in those who undergo steroid treatment

Questions

1. Which is not generally a finding of HSP?
   A. Gross hematuria
   B. Palpable purpura
   C. Arthritis of the knees
   D. Melena
   Answer: A

2. Which renal finding is uncommon with HSP?
   A. Red blood cell casts
   B. Peripheral edema
   C. Oliguria
   D. Proteinuria

   Answer: C

References

1. Bergstein J, Leiser J, Andreoli SP. Response of Crescentic Henoch-Schoenlein Purpura Nephritis to *Corticosteroid* and Azathioprine Therapy. *Clin Nephrol.* 1998 Jan; 49(1):9-14
2. Trapani S, Micheli A, Grisolia F, Resti M, Chiappini E, Falcini F, De Martino M. *Henoch Schonlein Purpura in Childhood: Epidemiological and Clinical Analysis of 150 Cases Over a 5-year Period and Review of Literature.* Semin Arthritis Rheum. 2005 Dec; 35(3):143-53.

Idiopathic Thrombocytopenia Purpura (ITP)

Critical Knowledge

Mental status changes or seizures in a child with ITP might signify intracranial hemorrhage—respond with immediate platelet transfusion and neurosurgical imaging and consultation

Background/Epidemiology/Anatomy

- Thrombocytopenia without identifiable cause and with no abnormalities of the bone marrow or other blood cell lines
- Incidence 50 per one million in the U.S.
- Two predominant forms with different natural histories
  - Acute ITP
    - Peaks at ages 2-4 years, no sex predominance
    - Often severe anemia, full recovery is the norm
    - Peaks in the winter and spring
  - Chronic ITP
    - Defined as having symptoms for over 6 months
    - More likely after age 10, twice as common in females
    - Generally insidious, worse long-term prognosis

Differential Diagnosis

- TTP/HUS
- Congenital thrombocytopenia purpura (e.g., Fanconi Syndrome, etc.)
- Infection (e.g., HIV and other viruses)
- Drugs (e.g., *heparin, sulfonamides, alcohol, quinidine*)
- Pseudothrombocytopenia secondary to EDTA use
- Liver disease
- Neonatal isoimmune thrombocytopenia
- Pregnancy
- Hypothyroidism
- Bone marrow infiltration (e.g., ALL, AML, myelofibrosis)

Critical Concepts

- Pathogenesis thought to be immunologic
  - Autoantibodies are thought to lead to platelet destruction
  - Megakaryocytes are generally normal or increased suggesting normal platelet formation
- ITP is a diagnosis of exclusion
- Physical exam may be normal
- Clinical signs/symptoms
  - General—children generally appear well
  - Hematologic—purpura and mucosal bleeding (often appear suddenly)
  - Gastrointestinal—no hepatosplenomegaly, occasional GI bleeding
  - Renal—hematuria
  - CNS—altered mental status from CNS hemorrhage (<1% of patients)
- Diagnostic findings
  - Thrombocytopenia—platelets normal in size and morphology
  - Normal INR/PT/PTT
  - No anemia or neutropenia (unless significant bleeding has occurred)
  - No evidence of hemolysis
  - Further studies
    - Imaging—CT head if intracranial bleeding suspected

        - When necessary—TSH, ANA, pregnancy testing, liver function panel, bone marrow aspirate

Treatment

- Supportive therapy
    - Stop exposure to medications which can cause thrombocytopenia
    - Encourage limitation of strenuous activity and contact sports
    - Blood transfusions
        - Platelets (1 unit/10 kg)—give only for on-going life-threatening bleeding, do not treat based on the level of thrombocytopenia
        - Packed-RBC's for anemia secondary to bleeding
- Observation alone appropriate for patients with minimal mucosal bleeding and platelet counts >30,000/mm^3
    - 80% of children will recover spontaneously in 4-8 weeks
- *Prednisone* (2 mg/kg/day)—does not alter time course of disease but will transiently increase platelets and decrease bleeding
- Intervenous immunoglobulin (IgG)(1 g/kg/dose IV)—single or multiple dose therapy will increase platelets
    - Appears more effective than *corticosteroids*
    - Consider pre-dosing *acetaminophen* and *diphenhydramine* to counteract side effects of headache, nausea and allergic reactions
- Anti-D(Rh) immunoglobulin (0.025-0.1 mg/kg)—similar effects as IgG administration
    - Only effective in Rh(+) patients
    - Side effect is hemolysis limiting its usefulness in anemic patients
- Splenectomy—effective treatment but used only for persistent and symptomatic thrombocytopenia
- Survival rate over 95%—most fatalities are from intracranial bleeding

Questions

1. Which is an inappropriate treatment for an asymptomatic child with ITP and a platelet count of 15,000/mm^3?
   A. Anti-D Immunoglobulin
   B. Intravenous Immunoglobulin (IgG)
   C. *Prednisone*
   D. Platelet transfusion
   Answer: D
2. Which would not be expected in a child with ITP and GI bleeding?
   A. Thrombocytopenia
   B. Decreased haptoglobin
   C. Normal INR/PT/PTT
   D. Anemia
   Answer: B

References

1. Ancona KG, Parker RI, Atlas MP, Prakash D. Randomized Trial of High-dose Methylprednisolone Versus Intravenous Immunoglobulin for the Treatment of Acute Idiopathic Thrombocytopenic Purpura in Children. *J Pediatr Hematol Oncol.* 2002 Oct; 24(7):540-4
2. Beck CE, Nathan PC, Parkin PC, Blanchette VS, Macarthur C. *Corticosteroids* Versus Intravenous Immune Globulin for the Treatment of Acute Immune Thrombocytopenic Purpura in Children: A Systematic Review and Meta-analysis of Randomized Controlled Trials. *J Pediatr.* 2005 Oct; 147(4):521-7.
3. Chu Y-W, Korb J, Sakamoto KM. Idiopathic Thrombocytopenic Purpura. *Pediatrics in Review.* 2000; 21:95-104.

Foreign Body Aspiration

Aaron Lessen, MD
Department of Emergency Medicine
The University of Arizona

Critical Knowledge

- Treatment of critical foreign body airway obstruction
    - If the patient can cough and make sounds, the foreign body airway obstruction is partial and no immediate intervention is needed
    - If the victim cannot cough or make any sound, the obstruction is severe and immediate intervention is necessary
        - For a child, perform subdiaphragmatic abdominal thrusts (Heimlich maneuver) until the object is expelled or the victim becomes unresponsive.
        - For an infant, deliver 5 back blows (slaps) with the infant in head-down position followed by 5 chest thrusts repeatedly until the object is expelled or the victim becomes unresponsive
        - If the victim becomes unresponsive, lay rescuers and healthcare providers should perform CPR but should look into the mouth before giving breaths, removing a foreign body if it is seen
        - If the obstruction persists, perform direct laryngoscopy to visualize and remove any foreign bodies using Magil forceps and perform endotracheal intubation as needed
        - If the foreign body cannot be removed and the patient cannot be ventilated, possible measures include pushing the foreign body into a main stem bronchus with an endotracheal tube, emergent consultation with anesthesia or a surgical service, needle cricothyroidotomy or emergent tracheostomy
- Maintaining a high index of suspicion for foreign body aspiration is essential, with close attention to history
    - Delayed diagnosis may lead to severe and possibly irreversible complications
    - A history suggestive of foreign body aspiration mandates endoscopic evaluation, regardless of radiological findings
        - Common signs and symptoms include choking, coughing, stridor, wheezing, respiratory distress or airway obstruction

- Lower airway symptoms may mimic asthma, croup, or URI, leading to frequent missed diagnoses
- Diagnostic studies include neck and chest radiographs, possibly fluoroscopy or virtual bronchoscopy
- Definitive diagnosis and treatment is rigid bronchoscopy performed by highly skilled personnel under general anesthesia

Epidemiology and Anatomy

- Foreign body obstruction of the upper airway can be immediately life threatening
- Causes 300 childhood deaths per year in the U.S., with 65% of victims less than 2 years old[2]
- 7% of lethal accidents in children aged 1-3[3]
- 60-80% of tracheobronchial foreign bodies occur in children less than 3 years[2]
- Serious complications from aspirated foreign bodies tend to occur in infants and younger children because of their small airway size[4]
- Male:female ratio usually reported as 2:1

Types of Foreign Bodies Aspirated

- Most foreign bodies are organic matter, with nuts and seeds accounting for 30% to 70% of cases, followed by other food products (apples, carrots, and popcorn), plants, and grasses
- Plastics and metals make up a minority of aspirated objects, and coin aspiration has rarely been reported
- Balloons are a toy that is commonly aspirated and can be deadly
- The severity of the foreign body aspiration is in part determined by the nature of the foreign body
- The majority of fatal accidents caused by a food-based foreign bodies are due to cylindrical or round foreign bodies that fit perfectly against the wall of the respiratory tract and cause asphyxia[1]
- Oil content in peanuts, seeds and nuts causes intense inflammatory responses[3]

Location of Foreign Body in the Respiratory Tree[4]

- Tracheal foreign bodies are uncommon (3–12% of foreign body aspirations)
- Foreign bodies are usually aspirated into one of the main bronchi, with the

right slightly more frequently involved than the left

- Foreign bodies have the potential for migration from one location to another
- Foreign bodies in the lower respiratory tree tend to have more non-specific symptoms and delayed presentation

Differential Diagnosis and Critical Concepts

- Differential diagnosis
  - Asthma
  - Pneumonia
  - Croup
  - Reactive airway diseases
  - Bronchiolitis
  - Epiglottitis
  - Larynigitis
  - Pulmonary lesions/disease
  - Upper respiratory infection
- High index of suspicion is essential
  - Sudden episode of coughing and choking or chronic, unexplained pulmonary infections should raise suspicion for foreign body aspiration
  - Wheezing (especially unilateral) in a patient without a history of asthma or other pulmonary disease should strongly suggest foreign body aspiration until proven otherwise
  - Early diagnosis prevents complications
- Signs and symptoms of foreign body aspiration are observed in three stages[4]
  - Initial stage
    - History of a choking episode – especially while eating or playing, followed by paroxysms of coughing or gagging
    - Initial symptoms include acute respiratory distress, stridor, increased respiratory effort, or complete obstruction
    - Physical exam findings include diminished breath sounds or wheezes from affected lung, but may be normal
    - A history of choking while holding or eating an object in the mouth is very predictive of foreign body aspiration

- The second stage is an asymptomatic interval
- The third stage is characterized by symptoms of delayed complications
  - Repeated or prolonged respiratory infections, wheezing refractory to conventional therapy, CXR findings

- Diagnostic Testing
  - PA and lateral CXR, soft tissue neck (AP, lateral)
    - CXR findings[6]
      - Hyperinflation or obstructive emphysema (range, 44-64%)
      - Mediastinal shift (range, 4-71%)
      - Pneumonia (range, 4-23%)
      - Atelectasis (range, 9-22%)
      - Radiopaque foreign body (range, 3-16%)
      - Unilateral whole-lung opacification (2%)
      - Normal (12-25%)
      - CXR findings not sensitive or specific
    - Differentiating tracheal and esophageal foreign bodies
      - Radiopaque FB in the trachea (such as a coin) will be seen on narrow edge on the PA CXR; FB in the esophagus will be seen on face in the PA CXR
  - Inspiratory and expiratory views may show unilateral air trapping
    - Lateral decubitus can be used in place of inspiration/expiration when patient cooperation is an issue
  - CT scan can be considered in cases of prolonged signs or symptoms to identify evidence of complications and possible radiopaque FB
  - Video fluoroscopy can be used to assess real time dynamic changes due to partial obstruction
  - Virtual bronchoscopy[7]
    - Noninvasive technique provides realistic 3D views of the tracheobronchial tree
    - Using a low-tube-current technique and rapid table speed can minimize radiation exposure
    - Can demonstrate both the foreign bodies in the airway and secondary parenchymal changes
    - Up to 100% sensitive and specific

    - Can be used to rule out FB and avoid unnecessary bronchoscopy (and potential complications) in lower suspicion cases with negative CXR
    - Can show the exact location of FB before bronchoscopy
- Diagnostic sensitivity of various signs or sypmtoms[8]
  - Choking crisis: sensitivity of 96% and a specificity of 76%
  - CXR: sensitivity of 70.3% and a specificity of 62.5%
  - Clinical examination: sensitivity of 84.2% and a specificity of 11.7%
  - Many patients are asymptomatic and have a normal CXR
  - No single sign, symptom or combination has been shown to be able to reliably confirm or exclude FBA (besides bronchoscopy)
- The diagnosis of foreign-body aspiration is often delayed
  - Studies suggest that early diagnosis within a day is made in only 60-70% of patients[2]
  - Diagnosis is delayed by one week in 8-33% of cases[1]
    - Delayed diagnosis associated with increased complications
    - One study showed that 75% of complications occurred in cases with delay of diagnosis of 24 hours
  - Many delayed diagnoses are related to reliance on a negative x-ray and are diagnosed as asthma or URI[4]
- Potential complications of foreign body aspiration[5]
  - Pneumomediastinum, pneumothorax, hydropneumothorax, bronchlal stenosis, abscess, atelectasis, pneumonia, bronchiectasis, foreign body dislodgment, and bronchospasm
- Suggested diagnostic strategy[2]
  - Obtain inspiratory and expiratory chest radiographs in all patients (or lateral decubitus)
  - With normal chest radiographs, a poor history for aspiration, and a patient with mild or no symptoms without focal findings on physical examination, the patient can be discharged with follow-up in a few days
  - If diagnosis remains unclear after plain films and there is a historical or clinical suspicion of aspiration, fluoroscopy may be obtained
  - When there is a high clinical index of suspicion (choking history with typically aspirated foods), bronchoscopy is indicated despite normal radiographic evaluation (including fluoroscopy)

        - May consider virtual or flexible bronchoscopy (when available) prior to rigid bronchoscopy

Treatment

- Initial First Aid (Pediatric Basic Life Support)
    - If the patient can cough and make some sounds, the airway obstruction is mild
        - Do not interfere, allow the patient to maintain a position of comfort
        - Allow the victim to clear the airway by coughing while you observe for signs of severe foreign body airway obstruction
    - If the victim cannot cough or make any sound, the airway obstruction is severe
        - For a child, perform subdiaphragmatic abdominal thrusts (Heimlich maneuver) until the object is expelled or the victim becomes unresponsive.
        - For an infant, deliver 5 back blows (slaps) with the infant in head-down position followed by 5 chest thrusts repeatedly until the object is expelled or the victim becomes unresponsive
            - Abdominal thrusts are not recommended for infants because they may damage the relatively large and unprotected liver
        - If the victim becomes unresponsive, lay rescuers and healthcare providers should perform CPR, but should look into the mouth before giving breaths
            - If a foreign body is seen, it should be removed
            - Healthcare providers should not perform blind finger sweeps because they may push obstructing objects further into the pharynx and may damage the oropharynx
            - If an object can be seen in the pharynx, healthcare providers should attempt to remove it and then rescuers should attempt ventilation, followed by chest compressions
    - Advanced Interventions[10]
        - If foreign body airway obstruction is not relieved with thrusts or compressions and condition deteriorates to respiratory failure or cardiopulmonary arrest, more aggressive interventions are necessary
        - Neutral, in-line positioning of the head, neck and shoulders and anterior displacement of the chin or jaw to facilitate an open mouth

- Perform direct laryngyscoy to visualize and remove the foreign with pediatric Magill forceps
  - Perfroming bag mask ventilation before attempting to remove the foreign body may worsen the obstruction
- If the foreign body cannot be seen in the pharynx or larynx, it may be in the esophagus, compressing the trachea
  - BLS maneuvers may dislodge the foreign body into the oropharynx where it can be removed
- If the foreign body is visualized in the subglottic space or trachea and cannot be removed, BLS maneuvers may dislodge it into the oropharynx
  - Alternatively, pushing the foreign body into a main stem bronchus with an endotracheal tube may allow ventilation of the other lung, but carries the risk of causing irreversible airway obstruction
- Emergent consultation with ENT, anesthesiology or general surgery is advisable at this point
- If above measures fail to clear the airway and the patient cannot be intubated or ventilated, emergency needle cricothyroidotomy is the procedure of last resort to provide oxygenation
  - Temporizing measure until definitive airway established
  - True complete airway obstruction is a relative contraindication to needle cricothyroidotomy as air cannot escape from the lungs, and an emergent tracheostomy may be more appropriate

- Bronchoscopy
  - Usually requires consultation with pediatric pulmonologists or pediatric surgeons
    - Most pulmonologists are not trained in rigid bronchoscopy and most are not trained in FB removal with flexible bronchoscopy
    - If only have access to personnel trained in diagnostic flexible bronchoscopy, may perform with a plan for transfer to facility with rigid bronchoscopy available
  - A history strongly suggestive for foreign body aspiration dictates diagnostic endoscopy with or without radiologic confirmation
  - Should be considered in cases with persistent respiratory signs and symptoms to rule out overlooked foreign body

- Flexible bronchoscopy is generally used for diagnostic purposes, not therapeutic
- Rigid bronchoscopy under general anesthesia is necessary for removal and is the treatment of choice
  - Grasping forceps or balloon tipped catheters can be used through bronchoscope for foreign body removal
  - Generally successful in removal of foreign body in 98% of cases, with rare need for thoracotomy
  - Can often be performed on outpatient basis, if no concern for respiratory status

- Flexible bronchoscopy has been used for FB removal in small studies[12]
  - Allows the retrieval of foreign bodies that have migrated deeper into the subsegmental bronchi that may be impossible to remove with rigid bronchoscope
- Potential complications of bronchoscopy
  - Pneumomediastinum, tracheal laceration, vocal cords laceration, sub-glottic edema, bronchospasm and necessity for thoracotomy, bronchotomy, or lobectomy (overall rate of complication low, 6-8%)[5]
  - Bronchoscopy should be performed by expertly trained personnel and the potential complications must be considered when deciding to perform bronchoscopy[11]
    - To avoid needless bronchoscopy, new imaging modalities such as virtual bronchoscopy may be considered
  - Complications are more likely in patients with delayed diagnosis (> 1 week since aspiration)[3]
- Education and prevention are the most important treatment
  - Should be aimed at increasing diagnostic acumen of the physicians and heightening of public awareness to reduce the morbidity and mortality
  - Parents should be instructed to abstain from feeding nuts and seeds to young children and to keep small, potentially ingestible objects out of their reach

Questions

1. Which of the following is true regarding the treatment of foreign body aspiration?

A. Bronchoscopy is only indicated when a foreign body is confirmed on radiographic testing

B. As soon as a patient starts choking after a suspected foreign body aspiration, abdominal thrusts should be performed to remove the foreign body

C. The rate of complications from bronchoscopy increase when the diagnosis is delayed more than one week

D. While performing CPR for the victim of a foreign body aspiration, blind finger sweeps should be made to retrieve a foreign body

E. Flexible bronchoscopy is widely accepted as the procedure of choice for removal of aspirated foreign bodies

Answer: C

2. You are evaluating a 2 year old patient who presents with sudden onset of coughing and mild respiratory distress. The child has no history of reactive airway disease. Which of the following is true regarding the diagnostic workup?

    A. Foreign body aspirations are rare in this age group and should not be suspected

    B. Inspiratory and expiratory view CXRs are indicated.

    C. If the patient has a normal CXR and a normal physical exam, a foreign body can be ruled out

    D. A radiopaque foreign body is likely to be found on CXR in cases of foreign body aspiration

    E. An initially missed diagnosis of foreign body aspiration does not lead to increased complication rates

    Answer: B

3. All of the following are true regarding pediatric foreign body aspirations except:

    A. Foreign body aspirations are more common in males

    B. Aspirated foreign bodies are most commonly organic food matter

    C. Foreign body aspirations are often misdiagnosed as asthma or respiratory infections

    D. Most aspirated foreign bodies settle in the left main stem bronchus

    E. Foreign bodies in the lower respiratory tree often have nonspecific symptoms and are delayed in diagnosis

    Answer: D

References

1. Rouillon I, Charrier JB, Devictor D, et al. Lower respiratory tract foreign bodies: a retrospective review of morbidity, mortality and first aid management. *Int J Pediatr Otorhinolaryngol.* 2006 Nov;70(11):1949-55.
2. Fleisher G, Ludwig S, Henreting F, eds. *Textbook of Pediatric Emergency Medicine.* Philadelphia, PA: Lippincott Williams & Wilkins, 2006.
3. Sersar S, Hamza UA, AbdelHameed WA, et al. Abstract Inhaled foreign bodies: management according to early or late presentation. *Eur J Cardiothorac Surg.* 2005 Sep;28(3):369-74.
4. Tan HK, Brown K, McGill T, et al. Airway foreign bodies (FB): a 10-year review. *Int J Pediatr Otorhinolaryngol.* 2000 Dec 1;56(2):91-9.
5. Oliveira CF, Almeida JF, Troster EJ, et al. Complications of tracheobronchial foreign body aspiration in children: report of 5 cases and review of the literature. *Rev Hosp Clin Fac Med Sao Paulo.* 2002 May-Jun;57(3):108-11.
6. Girardi G, Contador AM, Castro-Rodriguez JA. Two new radiological findings to improve the diagnosis of bronchial foreign-body aspiration in children. *Pediatr Pulmonol.* 2004 Sep;38(3):261-4.
7. Kosucu P, Ahmetoglu A, Koramaz I, et al. Low-dose MDCT and virtual bronchoscopy in pediatric patients with foreign body aspiration. *AJR Am J* Roentgenol. 2004 Dec;183(6):1771-7.
8. Metrangelo S, Monetti C, Meneghini L, et al. Eight years' experience with foreign-body aspiration in children: what is really important for a timely diagnosis? *J Pediatr Surg.* 1999 Aug;34(8):1229-31.
9. 2005 American Heart Association Guidelines for Cardiopulmonary Resuscitation and Emergency Cardiovascular Care, Part 11: Pediatric Basic Life Support. Circulation 2005;112;156-166.
10. Marx, J ed. Rosen's Emergency Medicine: Concepts and Clinical Practice, 6th ed. Philadelphia, PA: Mosby, 2006.
11. Ciftci AO, Bingol-Kologlu M, Senocak ME, et al. Bronchoscopy for evaluation of foreign body aspiration in children. *J Pediatr Surg.* 2003 Aug;38(8):1170-6.
12. Swanson KL, Prakash UB, Midthun DE, et al. Flexible bronchoscopic management of airway foreign bodies in children. Chest. 2002 May;121(5):1695-700.

Foreign Body Ingestion

Aaron Lessen, MD
Department of Emergency Medicine
The University of Arizona

Critical Knowledge

- FB ingestion rarely causes immediately life threatening complications
- Very common pediatric problem, especially in 6 months to 3 years age group
- Physicians must keep a high index of suspicion for foreign body ingestion in cases of witnessed ingestion or with suggestive symptoms such as gagging, vomiting, dysphagia, refusal to eat, wheezing or foreign body sensation
- Retained ingested foreign bodies may lead to potentially serious complications, including respiratory distress, perforation, obstruction and possibly death. The longer foreign bodies are impacted, the more likely complications become
- Many foreign body ingestions are asymptomatic and the foreign body often passes with no complications or symptoms
- Diagnostic tests include radiographs and possibly contrast esophagram
- Treatment of foreign bodies lodged in the esophagus includes immediate removal versus observation period of up to 24 hours [in asymptomatic patients with acute (<24 hrs) FB ingestion] for spontaneous passage
- Disc batteries that lodge in the esophagus should be removed emergently because of the potential to rapidly injure the esophagus
- Once foreign bodies advance past the esophagus, they often will pass through the GI tract spontaneously, but debate exists for treatment of long and sharp objects

Epidemiology and Anatomy

- FB ingestions are extremely common
    - 182,105 incidents of foreign body ingestion in 1999 in patients younger than 20 years as reported by the American Association of Poison Control in 1999.[1]
    - 5-10% of children reported to have swallowed a coin at some point.[2]
- Typical age of presentation is 6 months to 3 years, with boys more common than girls
- Ingested foreign bodies may lodge in the esophagus or may be unable to pass through more distal portions of the GI tract including the pylorus,

duodenum, cecum, appendix, or rectum

- Impaction in the esophagus is the most common and potentially the most serious
  - 70% of esophageal foreign bodies become lodged at the thoracic inlet
    - The superior esophagus is the narrowest portion of the pediatric GI tract
    - The location of the circopharyngeus sling (C6)
  - 15% become impacted at the level of the aortic arch
  - 15% become impacted at the gastroesophageal junction

- Nature of ingested pediatric foreign bodies
  - Most childhood esophageal foreign bodies are round or spherical
  - Coins are the most common foreign body ingested and make up 50% to 75% of childhood esophageal foreign bodies. Pennies are the most common coin ingested.
  - Children are less likely than adults to have foodstuffs foreign bodies in the esophagus
  - Fish bone ingestions are especially common in children in Asian communities
  - Children with anatomic or physiologic esophageal or GI tract abnormalities are more likely to suffer foreign body impaction
- Foreign bodies that reach the stomach safely will usually traverse the remainder of the GI tract without complications
  - Some studies suggest that up to 85% of coin ingestions are managed safely at home with no physician evaluation or interventions, with no complications.[2]
  - A variety of foreign bodies, including screws, tacks and staples, have been documented to traverse the entire GI tract safely
  - Some objects longer than 5 cm or greater than 2 cm in diameter may not be able to safely pass through the tight turns of the duodenum and other portions of the lower GI tract
  - Some very sharp objects such as sewing needles or toothpicks have higher risk of perforating hollow viscera. Bowel perforation from sharp objects has resulted in peritonitis, abscess formation, inflammatory tumors, hemorrhage, and death

Differential Diagnosis and Critical Concepts

- Differential diagnosis
  - Foreign body aspiration
  - Esophagitis
  - GERD
  - Gastritis
  - Peptic ulcer disease
  - Reactive airway disease
  - Pharyngitis
  - Esophageal stricture
  - Gastroenteritis
  - Munchausen syndrome
  - Obstruction, large or small bowel
  - Intussusception
  - Pyloric stenosis
  - Aspiration pneumonia
  - Pneumomediastinum
  - Acute appendicitis
  - Psychiatric diseases - autism, bulimia, mental retardation, personality disorders
- Adverse effects and symptoms usually result from esophageal impaction
  - Symptoms of esophageal impaction include gagging, vomiting, drooling, (possibly coughing) dysphagia, refusal to eat, foreign body sensation, pain, localization, wheezing, or generalized irritability
  - Symptoms with a history of swallowing a FB make the diagnosis straightforward
  - When there is no definite history of FB ingestion, the diagnosis of a FB can be difficult as the symptoms may mimic other common childhood conditions
  - Impacted esophageal foreign bodies may induce secondary airway symptoms
  - May be asymptomatic (30-40% of patients with esophageal coins)

- Symptoms relating to serious complications
  - Esophageal perforation: neck swelling, crepitations, and pneumomediastinum.
  - Stomach or GI perforation: fever, abdominal pain and tenderness
  - Bowel obstruction: abdominal distension, pain, and tenderness
- Diagnostic approach[4]
  - If there is a history of suggested FB ingestion, perform radiographic evaluation (CXR and soft tissue neck, possible abdominal XR)
    - Asymptomatic patient who has ingested a small (less than 1 cm in maximum diameter), nonsharp object may not require imaging studies
    - Radiopaque FB found in approximately 65% of cases
- Differentiating tracheal and esophageal foreign bodies
  - Radiopaque FB in the trachea (such as a coin) will be seen on narrow edge on the PA CXR; FB in the esophagus will be seen on face in the PA CXR
- If the foreign body is not radiopaque but is large enough to become impacted, such as a large food bolus, and the symptoms suggest esophageal impaction, obtain either a contrast esophagram or immediate endoscopy. Esophagrams pose risk of aspiration and make subsequent endoscopy more difficult.
- Handheld metal detectors can provide a diagnostic alternative to radiography as initial screen when a coin ingestion is suspected.[5]
  - Compared favorably with radiography in determining presence or absence of a coin and coin location (esophagus or more distal GI tract)
  - Patient follow-up is suggested because esophageal coins may be missed (especially in obese children)
- Missed foreign body ingestion with retained FB can occasionally lead to serious sequelae, including bronchoesophageal fistula, mediastinitis, esophageal diverticulum, lobar atelectasis, aortoesophageal fistula and need for thoracotomy for FB removal

Treatment

- Oropharyngeal foreign bodies
  - Can usually be identified and removed by a number of methods
  - Forceps and tongue depressor, transnasal flexible endosopy, direct laryngoscopy and indirect laryngoscopy have all been used successfully.[6]

- Esophageal foreign bodies
    - Sharp esophageal foreign bodies and disc batteries should be removed promptly
        - Disc batteries may cause esophageal injury within hours that can lead to permanent sequelae and should be removed emergently
    - Observation for spontaneous passage is a possible option [9]
        - Most likely to occur when the object is lodged at the gastroesophageal junction, but is also possible with coins in proximal or mid esophagus
        - Observation with spontaneous passage avoids costs and potential complications of removal techniques
        - Reasonable to allow a period of 12 to 24 hours for spontaneous passage
            - General criteria for observation
                - Round, noncorrosive (e.g., coins) foreign bodies
                - Asymptomatic patient (i.e., no respiratory distress)
                - No history of esophageal disease
                - Ingestion occurred less than 24 hours prior
            - No complications have been reported during 24 hour observation period (at home or hospital admission for observation)
        - Randomized prospective study of immediate endoscopic removal of esophageal coins compared to 16 hour observation in 60 patients [7]
            - Spontaneous passage occurred equally in observation group and surgical group (25%)
            - Spontaneous passage more likely in older patients (66 vs 46 months), male patients, and coins in distal 1/3 of esophagus
            - No complications in either group
        - Coins throughout the esophagus have been shown to have good spontaneous passage rate in 12-24 hour observation period[9], 22% of proximal, 33% middle, 37% distal coins
        - Observation period should only be attempted with good follow-up and after consultation with the physician who will be involved in the potential removal
        - No serious complications have been documented from an

esophageal coin that was impacted for less than a few days. However, the esophageal mucosa may grow around a coin after several days, making removal more difficult.

- Removal techniques
  - Techniques vary regionally and depend on the duration of impaction, associated symptoms, and the nature of the foreign body
  - Traditional removal methods include rigid esophagoscopy under general anesthesia, and flexible endoscopy under sedation
    - Esophagoscopy under general anesthesia has been the method of choice for many years. Proven to be safe and efficacious, is applicable to all types of foreign bodies, allows for direct examination of the esophageal lumen, and can be used in patients with respiratory distress.
    - Possible but rare complications of endoscopy or esophagoscopy include pharyngeal bleeding, bronchospasm, accidental extubation, stridor, hypoxia, esophageal perforation, and mediastinitis[7]
    - Immediate endoscopic removal is still essential in patients not meeting criteria for observation or alternative removal techniques
  - Direct laryngoscopy with or without sedation can be diagnostic and therapeutic for coins in the upper esophagus and non-metallic small objects (such as bones)
  - For coins and similar round, smooth objects, several alternative methods have been developed
    - Strict selection criteria for alternative techniques
      - Single foreign body ingestion
      - Acute ingestion (less than 24 hours)
      - Child with no history of esophageal abnormalities and no previous foreign body ingestion
      - No respiratory distress
      - No evidence of esophageal perforation or other serious complication
    - Balloon-tipped catheter under fluoroscopic guidance to extract or advance the coin

            - Success rate of approximately 90% (extraction or advancing FB into stomach)
            - Higher failure rates in younger children (< 2 years)
            - Significant cost savings compared to rigid esophagoscopy
            - Has been criticized because of lack of airway control, poor control of the foreign body during extraction, and inadequate visualization of the esophagus. Complications are rare (~ 2%) and include epistaxis, vomiting, respiratory distress, esophageal perforation
        - Bougienage to advance the coin into the stomach
            - When used selectively has a high success rate and very safe with few complications at several institutions
            - Much less costly than esophagoscopy with general anesthesia
            - Has been used by trained emergency physicians safely and effectively[8]
        - Fluoroscopic-guided grasping endoscopic forceps covered by a soft rubber catheter takes only 1 minute, but experience is limited
    - Medications
        - Medications such as *gulcagon* or *diazepam* have been used to facilitate the passage of foreign bodies from the esophagus by reducing muscular tone, enhancing esophageal motility, or relaxing the lower esophageal sphincter
        - Success with these methods is mostly anecdotal, and there are few studies comparing the use of medications with spontaneous passage rates
        - Recent small double blinded placebo controlled study showed that *glucagon* did not increase the rate of spontaneous esophageal coin passage when compared to placebo[10]
- Stomach and lower GI foreign bodies
    - Can usually be managed expectantly
    - Management recommendations for sharp objects are varied but conservative—watchful waiting is usually safe
        - Sewing needles have increased propensity for perforation, and should probably be removed

        - Long objects (greater than 3-5 cm in children >1 year, 2 cm under 1 year) should also be removed from the stomach
        - A recent expert panel recommended that large or sharp objects be removed endoscopically before they have passed beyond the duodenal curve because they are more likely to cause complications or require surgical removal [11]
            - If cannot be removed, recommend daily radiographs and surgical removal if no progression in 3 days
    - Most round objects (e.g., coins) will traverse the GI tract in 3 to 8 days without any complication, but some may take up to 4 weeks
    - Some objects remain in the stomach for a long duration
        - Weekly radiographs for progression
        - Three to four weeks should be allowed for passage of inert objects out of the stomach before surgical or endoscopic removal is necessary
        - Removal should be considered for objects in same position for more than one week or with any fever, vomiting, abdominal pain, or other significant symptoms
    - Some physicians advocate parental examination of the stool for the foreign body
        - In practice this may not be very useful
        - Unpleasant task that is commonly abandoned
- Disc battery ingestion
    - Disc batteries that lodge in the esophagus should be removed emergently because of the potential to rapidly injure the esophagus from corrosive effects
    - Disc batteries that pass the esophagus safely and spontaneously can be observed
        - Batteries should be removed endoscopically if they remain in the stomach for more than 48 hours or are larger than 2 cm in diameter
        - Once batteries are past the duodenal sweep, 85 percent pass in less than 72 hours
        - Radiographs should be obtained every three to four days to follow the progress until it has passed, unless symptoms develop

    - Only sporadic cases of systemic absorption of battery contents have been suggested in the literature, and no serious toxicities have been reported
- Prevention of FB ingestion is the best treatment, with efforts targeted to preschool toddler group
    - Appropriate foods and supervised play

Questions

1. Which of the following is true regarding pediatric foreign body ingestions?
    A. Foreign body ingestions are rare and usually cause immediate life-threatening symptoms
    B. Most ingested foreign bodies become impacted at the gastroesohageal junction
    C. Most foreign bodies that reach the stomach safely will traverse the remainder of the GI tract without complications
    D. Most foreign body impactions are a result of large food boluses
    E. Girls are more likely to have a foreign body ingestion

    Answer: C

2. Which of the following is not an accepted criteria for observation of an esophageal foreign body?
    A. Round, noncorrosive foreign bodies
    B. Patients must be hospitalized during observation period
    C. No history of esophageal disease
    D. Asymptomatic patient
    E. Ingestion occurred less than 24 hours prior

    Answer: B

3. Which of the following is true when managing a GI tract foreign body?
    A. All objects larger than 1 cm in diameter should be removed, regardless of their location
    B. Medications such as *glucagon* have been proven to be highly effective in advancing foreign bodies through the GI tract
    C. Rigid esophagoscopy is the only acceptable method of removing esophageal foreign bodies
    D. The spontaneous passage rate of coins from the esophagus is approximately 30%

E. If foreign bodies are observed for spontaneous passage, thorough stool inspection is mandatory

Answer: D

References

1. Wong KK, Fang CX, Tam PK. Selective upper endoscopy for foreign body ingestion in children: an evaluation of management protocol after 282 cases. *J Pediatr Surg.* 2006 Dec;41 (12):2016-8.
2. Conners GP, Chamberlain JM, Weiner PR. Pediatric coin ingestion: a home-based survey. *Am J Emerg Med.* 1995 Nov;13 (6):638-40.
3. Conners GP, Cobaugh DJ, Feinberg, et al. Home observation for asymptomatic coin ingestion: acceptance and outcomes. The New York State Poison Control Center Coin Ingestion Study Group. *Acad Emerg Med.* 1999 Mar;6 (3):213-7.
4. Fleisher G, Ludwig S, Henreting F, eds. *Textbook of Pediatric Emergency Medicine.* Philadelphia, PA: Lippincott Williams & Wilkins, 2006.
5. Bassett KE, Schunk JE, Logan L. Localizing ingested coins with a metal detector. *Am J Emerg Med.* 1999 Jul;17 (4):338-41.
6. Wai Pak M, Chung Lee W, Kwok Fung H, et al. A prospective study of foreign-body ingestion in 311 children. *Int J Pediatr Otorhinolaryngol.* 2001 Apr 6;58 (1):37-45.
7. Waltzman ML, Baskin M, Wypij D. A randomized clinical trial of the management of esophageal coins in children. *Pediatrics.* 2005 Sep;116 (3):614-9.
8. Emslander HC, Bonadio W, Klatzo M. Efficacy of esophageal bougienage by emergency physicians in pediatric coin ingestion. *Ann Emerg Med.* 1996 Jun;27 (6):726-9.
9. Soprano JV, Fleisher GR, Mandl KD. *The spontaneous passage of esophageal coins in children.* Arch Pediatr Adolesc Med. 1999 Oct;153 (10):1073-6.
10. Mehta D, Attia M, Quintana E *Glucagon* use for esophageal coin dislodgment in children: a prospective, double-blind, placebo-controlled trial. *Acad Emerg Med.* 2001 Feb;8 (2):200-3.
11. Eisen GM, Baron TH, Dominitz JA et al. *Guideline for the management of ingested foreign bodies.* Gastrointest Endosc. 2002 Jun;55 (7):802-6.

Hyperbilirubinemia

Scott Thielen, MD, MS
Department of Emergency Medicine
University of Minnesota
James Colletti, MD, FACEP
Assistant Professor
Department of Emergency Medicine
University of Minnesota

Neonatal (Jaundice)

Background

Definition

Jaundice is a yellowish-greenish pigmentation of the sclera and/or skin caused by deposition of bilirubin.

Diagnosis

Serum bilirubin >5 mg/dl, yellowish pigment in sclera, blanching the skin to look at underlying pigment.

Pathophysiology

A. Three general causes of hyperbilirubinemia
   1. Increased production of unconjugated bilirubin
   2. Inability of immature liver to conjugate bilirubin
   3. Liver cannot uptake bilirubin (occurs in Gilbert's Syndrome)

B. Bilirubin forms
   1. Unconjugated bilirubin = indirect bilirubin
      - Toxic breakdown product of hemoglobin
      - Difficult to excrete but able to cross the blood brain barrier into central nervous system resulting in kernicterus
      - Liver makes it conjugated bilirubin with enzyme UDPGT
   2. Conjugated bilirubin = direct bilirubin
      - Non toxic and easy to excrete because water soluble
      - Unable to cross the blood brain barrier

    - Eliminated in stool but can be broken down by bacteria to unconjugated bilirubin then reabsorbed back into blood stream (enterohepatic circulation)
  3. Total bilirubin = conjugated and unconjugated forms

Risk Factors

A. Jaundice present in first 24 hours

B. Jaundice develops before hospital discharge

C. Hx of jaundiced sibling

D. Early gestation <38 weeks

E. Exclusive breast feeding

F. East Asian race

G. Bruising, cephalohematoma, or hemolysis

H. Maternal age >or equal to 25 year old

I. Male sex

Signs of Pathologic Jaundice

A. First 24 hours of life

B. Rapidly rising serum bilirubin (>5 mg/dL per day)

C. In the presence of anemia or hepatosplenomegaly

A. Prolonged jaundice (>7 to 10 days in a full-term infant)

B. Elevated direct bilirubin concentration (>2 mg/dL or >20% of total serum bilirubin)

Differential Diagnosis by Etiology

Unconjugated Hyperbilirubinemia

A. Increased bilirubin load

  1. Fetal-maternal blood group incompatibility
  2. Autoimmune hemolytic anemia
  3. G6PD (occurs in about 12% of African-Americans; common in Mediterranean, Middle East, Africa and SE Asia)
  4. Abnormality of the red blood cell membrane
  5. Hematoma, occult hemorrhage, or polycythemia
  6. Sepsis with hemolysis
  7. Medications

8. Physiologic jaundice: breakdown of fetal RBC's and hepatocytes can't handle unconjugated bilirubin yet

B. Decreased bilirubin excretion/uptake

1. Delay in intestinal transit time
2. Crigler-Najjar Syndrome (Type I: extreme jaundice with bilirubin >25 mg/dL, high risk of bilirubin encephalopathy; Type II: treatment is with *phenobarbital*)
3. Neonatal hypothyroidism
4. Breast milk jaundice
   - Breast milk feeding is associated with neonatal hyperbilirubinemia
   - For healthy newborns the danger is minimal and switching to formula is unnecessary

Conjugated Hyperbilirubinemia

A. Lacks toxicity but is a marker for a serious underlying disease

B. Hepatitis

C. Cholestasis

D. Cystic fibrosis

E. Sepsis (CMV, TORCH infections, Hep B) usually presents with other signs (i.e., vomiting, abdominal distention, respiratory distress, and poor feeding)

F. Inborn error of metabolism

G. Inflammation

H. Mass lesion

I. Generally present with clinical jaundice in the first 4 weeks of life

<u>Complications</u>: kernicterus is a rare but catastrophic bilirubin induced brain injury

Emergency Medicine Implications

Emergency Department Evaluation

A. Full H&P looking especially at extent of jaundice, neurologic abnormalities, vitals

B. Labs: measure total, direct and indirect bilirubin, U/A, CBC

1. Concern for sepsis: above and blood cx, urine cx, CSF studies, stool cx, TORCH panel, hepatitis B serologies, urine for CMV

2. Hemolysis: Coombs test, haptoglobin, smear maternal and fetal ABO types
3. Others etiologies
    - Consider complete LFTs (AST, ALT, alk phos, ammonia, albumin, total protein, coagulation studies) if mostly direct bilirubinemia
    - Basic metabolic panel
    - Urine for reducing substances
    - Consider: alpha 1 antitrypsin, sweat chloride, red blood cell galactose-1-phosphate uridyltransferase
    - Check G-6-PD if poor response to phototherapy or clinical suspicion
4. If biliary atresia or obstruction is a concern: abdominal ultrasonography

C. Decision making
1. Infant is well appearing, afebrile with unconjugated hyperbilirubinemia and normal hemoglobin, no further labs
2. Further workup for concern of sepsis, hemolysis, inborn errors of metabolism
3. Plot infant on Table 1 and 2 below with possible admit for further workup and phototherapy

Emergency Department Treatment

A. Goal to identify and treat threats to life (i.e., sepsis) and risk stratify

B. Dehydration: correct dehydration with normal *saline* boluses
1. Frequent feeds and frequent stools help excrete bilirubin
2. Options for feeding with or without phototherapy
    - Continuation of breast feeding with close monitoring
    - Supplementation with formula
    - Brief interruption of breast feeding and substitution of formula
    - In cases of breast milk jaundice, consider temporary cessation of breast milk with re-introduction after the bilirubin has fallen to a safe level

C. Phototherapy
1. A blue light that causes photoconversion of the bilirubin molecule to a water-soluble product that is excreted in the urine and stool

2. May lead to greater water loss
   - Fluid intake must be increased by 20%
   - Breast feeding may be continued
3. Rules for starting phototherapy: use Table 1 to determine if phototherapy needed

D. Exchange transfusion
1. Emergent treatment for markedly elevated bilirubin with signs of bilirubin encephalopathy.
2. Exchange transfusion is recommended for term infants with hemolysis, if phototherapy is unable to maintain the total bilirubin level below 17.5 – 23.4 mg/dL.

E. Correction of anemia secondary to isoimmune hemolytic disease
1. Reduces the bilirubin concentration by approximately 50%
2. Should be used with concurrent phototherapy

F. Treat underlying disorder if able

G. Consider admission depending on bilirubin level, need for phototherapy, whether further workup is needed, and for certain pathology that needs close monitoring (sepsis, ABO incompatibility, etc.)

H. Future directions in therapy: medications to block bilirubin production from hemoglobin (*tin-mesoporphyrin* is in clinical trials currently)

Kernicterus (Bilirubin Encephalopathy)

Definition

Encephalopathy due to accumulation of unconjugated bilirubin in the brain

Diagnosis

Unconjugated hyperbilirubinemia and clinical signs of neurologic compromise

Clinical Picture

Initially manifests as seizure, lethargy, poor suck and feeding poorly with evidence of jaundice. Differentiate this from botulism by jaundice. Later findings include hypertonicity, fever and high-pitched cry. The baby can have retrocollis (arching of neck backwards) or opisthotonus (backwards arching of trunk). The hypertonicity can also be seen in infant C. tetani infection. Chronic manifestations of kernicterus include extrapyramidal movement disorders, athetoid cerebral palsy, spasticity, gaze abnormalities, weakness, hearing difficulties and mental retardation.

Pathophysiology

Unconjugated bilirubin is directly toxic to brain cells. Basal ganglia and brainstem nuclei appear to be more susceptible than other areas of the brain. This toxicity is manifested in the signs listed above.

Emergency Department Management

(Please see section on hyperbilirubinemia for a complete discussion)

A. Any infant with hyperbilirubinemia and signs of encephalopathy (see above) needs immediate exchange transfusion in a neonatal intensive care unit.

B. In isoimmune hemolytic disease, can use intravenous γ-globulin (0.5-1 g/kg over 2 hours) if the TSB continues to rise even with phototherapy or the total bilirubin is within 2 to 3 mg/dL of the level requiring an exchange transfusion. The initial dose can be repeated once in 12 hours if needed.

C. Please see Table 1 for phototherapy and Table 2 for exchange transfusion in hyperbilirubinemia section.

D. Workup to determine cause of hyperbilirubinemia: see section on hyperbilirubinemia

Table 1: Total Bilirubin Levels and Phototherapy Initiation

	Hours From Birth						
	Birth	12	24	48	72	96	>96
High Risk	>4	>6	>8	>11	>13.5	>14.5	>15
Medium Risk	>5	>7.5	>9.5	>13	>15	>17	>18
Low Risk	>7	>9	>11.5	>15	>17.5	>20	>21

Total Serum Bilirubin (mg/dl)

(NOTE: low risk implies gestation >38 weeks and well, medium risk >38 weeks and risk factors, and high risk 35-38 weeks gestation and risk factors. The above table is not applicable to gestations <35 weeks.)

Table 2: Level to Initiate Exchange Transfusion

	Hours From Birth						
	Birth	12	24	48	72	96	>96
High Risk	>12	>13	>15	>17	>18.5	>19	>19
Medium Risk	>14	>15	>16.5	>19	>21	>22	>22
Low Risk	>16	>17.5	>19	>22	>24	>25	>25

Total Serum Bilirubin (mg/dl)

(NOTE: low risk implies gestation >38 weeks and well, medium risk >38 weeks and risk factors, and high risk 35-38 weeks gestation and risk factors. The above table is not applicable to gestations <35 weeks.)

Questions

1. Which of the following is not consistent with pathologic jaundice?
   A. Jaundice within the first 24 hours of life
   A. Slow rising serum bilirubin
   B. Prolonged jaundice (>7 to 10 days in a full term infant)
   C. Elevated direct bilirubin level (>2 mg/dl)u

   Answer: B
2. Which of the following are NOT in the differential diagnosis of unconjugated hyperbilirubinemia?
   A. Sepsis with hemolysis
   B. Physiologic jaundice
   C. Cystic fibrosis
   D. Crigler-Najjar Syndrome

   Answer: C
3. A 6 day old infant is brought to your Emergency Room for poor feeding. She was born via an uncomplicated vaginal delivery. There were no complications of the mothers prenancy nor delivery. On physical exam you note that the child is jaundiced. The child appears lethargic and has increased tone in her extremitics. Appropriate management for this child should include all of the following except
   A. Admission to the neonatal intensive care unit
   B. Sepsis workup
   C. Immediate initiation of exchange transfusion
   D. Phototherapy
   E. Discharge to home

   Answer: E

References

1. American Academy of Pediatrics Subcommittee on Hyperbilirubinemia. Management of hyperbilirubinemia in the newborn infant 35 or more weeks of gestation. *Pediatrics*. 114(1):297-316, 2004 Jul.
2. Bhutani VK, D. S., Johnson LH (2005). *Risk Management of Severe Neonatal Hyperbilirubinemia to Prevent Kernicterus*. Clin Perinatol 32(1): 125-39.
3. Brown, A. (1962). *Neonatal Jaundice*. Pediatr Clin of North Am 9: 589.
4. Claudius I, F. C., Boles R (2005). *The Emergency Department Approach to Newborn and Childhood Metabolic Crisis*. Emerg Med Clin N Am 23: 843-883.
5. Dennery PA. Metalloporphyrins for the treatment of neonatal jaundice. Current Opinion in Pediatrics. 17(2):167-9, 2005 Apr.
6. Dennery PA, S. D. S., Stevenson DK (2001). Neonatal Hyperbilirubinemia. *N Engl J Med* 344(8): 581 - 590.
7. Huang MJ, K. K., Teng HC, Tang KS, Weng HW, Huang CS (2004). *Risk Factors for Severe Hyperbilirubinemia in Neonates*. Pediatr Res 56(5): 682-9.
8. Ip S. Chung M. Kulig J. O'Brien R. Sege R. Glicken S. Maisels MJ. Lau J. (American Academy of Pediatrics Subcommittee on Hyperbilirubinemia). An evidence-based review of important issues concerning neonatal hyperbilirubinemia. *Pediatrics*. 114(1):e130-53, 2004 Jul.
9. Table 1: Total Bilirubin Levels and Phototherapy Initiation, Adapted from: Fig 3. Guidelines for phototherapy in hospitalized infants of 35 or more weeks' gestation. *Pediatrics* Vol. 114 No. 1 July 2004, pp. 297-316.
10. Table 2: Level to Initiate Exchange Transfusion, Adapted from Fig 4. Guidelines for exchange transfusion in infants 35 or more weeks' gestation. *Pediatrics* Vol. 114 No. 1 July 2004, pp. 297-316

Neurologic Emergencies

Barrett Adams, MD
Department of Emergency Medicine
North Sound Emergency Medicine, Everett, WA

Seizure

Critical Knowledge

- ABC's, IV, monitor, oxygen, blood *glucose*
- Consider eliciting event
- Status epilepticus: *benzodiazepines*, then consider *phenobarbital* or *phenytoin*

Background

Seizure is a relatively common presenting complaint in pediatric emergency department visits, with approximately 4-6% of the population suffering a seizure by age 16. **S**tatus **E**pilepticus (**SE**) is traditionally defined as seizure, or of multiple seizures without return to baseline with a duration longer than 30 minutes. 30% of epileptics will present initially in SE. A true emergency, timely efforts need to be made to control both clinical as well as electrical, seizure activity. Increased neuronal damage in SE appears correlated with younger age, generalized seizures, and longer duration, and shows injury patterns similar to cerebral hypoxia.

Classification of Seizures

Partial (focal involvement of brain)
• Simple – no loss of consciousness
• Complex – impairment in consciousness
  ► Temporal lobe (change in consciousness only)
  ► Generalizing (progress to tonic-clonic)

Generalized (involve majority of cerebral cortex) • Absence – brief loss of awareness • Tonic – muscle contraction and rigidity • Clonic – jerking and spasm • Tonic – clonic • Myoclonic – brief muscle contractions • Atonic – loss of all muscle tone

Differential/Critical Concepts

The most common etiology of seizures in children is fever, although this is a diagnosis of exclusion, considering other causes based on age and co-morbidities. For patients who are taking anti-seizure medications, being sub-theraputic or simple withdrawal is a common cause of seizures.

Potential Seizure Etiologies Based on Age
Neonatal: hypoxia, drugs, trauma, infection, hypo/hyperglycemia, *pyridoxine* deficiency, drug withdrawal, inborn errors of metabolism, hyper/hyponatremia
0-6 months: infection, hypocalcemia, hyperphosphatemia, hyponatremia, developmental malformation, inborn error of metabolism
6 months-3 years: fever, infection, toxin, trauma, metabolic disorder
Over 3 years: idiopathic, infection, trauma, sleep deprivation, mass

Treatment and Work-up

General principles

- ABC's and D! (D = dextrose)
- Maintain oxygenation and airway
- Check *glucose*
- Establish IV access
- Protecting child from further harm (seizure pads, remove obstacles)

Status Epilepticus

- *Benzodiazepines* - 80% effective in controlling SE
- Second line antiepileptics,
  - *Phenobarbital* - (20 mg/kg IV, IM)
  - *Fosphenytoin* - (20 *phenytoin* equivalents/kg IV, IM)
  - *Phenytoin* - (20 mg/kg IV) **SLOW!**
- If refractory, consider intubation and sedation with *Propofol* or *barbiturates*
- EEG monitoring
- Work up considerations
  - Head CT
  - Blood *glucose*
  - Chemistry panel
  - Therapeutic drug levels

- CBC
- Toxicology screen
- Urinalysis
- In the neonatal period consider *pyridoxine* in the refractory seizure

Febrile Seizure

Critical Knowledge

Self limited relatively common event in the febrile child

Background

Febrile seizures are the most common seizure event observed in the young pediatric population. It is estimated approximately 5% of children will experience a febrile seizure. In its most common form, a simple febrile seizure is self limited and benign, requiring only supportive measures and no extensive diagnostic evaluation, aside from that normally performed for a fever in the respective age group and co-morbid state. A complex febrile seizure may be associated a more severe pathology and requires more extensive evaluation.

Simple Febrile Seizure

- Fever present
- Generalized convulsions
- Last less than 15 minutes
- Do not re-occur within 24 hrs

Complex Febrile Seizure

- Lasts more than 15 minutes or
- Re-occurs within 24 hrs or
- Has a focal component

Differential/Critical Concepts

Most febrile seizures occur between the ages of 9 months to 3 years, with range from 3 months to 5 years. Febrile seizures have a strong familial component and are associated with a slightly higher lifetime risk of epilepsy, estimated to be 2% versus 1% in the general population. The risk for a febrile seizure does not appear to be correlated with rise in temperature, although does appear to have a relation to high fever. Thirty percent of children will have a recurrent febrile seizure in a subsequent illness. The differential must include consideration of trauma, toxic ingestions, or meningitis. Risks of meningitis include: a doctor visit within the previous 48 hours, seizure activity at presentation to the ED, focal seizures, concerning physical exam findings, or an abnormal neurologic exam.

Treatment and Work-up

Febrile seizures are given a very narrow definition since, by making the diagnosis, the examining physician is essentially declaring that no underlying CNS pathology exists. The extent of workup for a child presenting to the ED with a febrile seizure will vary greatly based on the clinical picture and circumstances at hand. In 1996, the AAP published practice parameters for the management of acute febrile seizures. Table 1 outlines the AAP's guidelines for the neurodiagnostic evaluation of a child with a simple febrile seizure between the ages of 6 months and 5 years. In the absence of suspicious history such as vomiting, diarrhea, or concerning physical exam findings, CBC, electrolytes or blood *glucose* are of limited value in the examination of child greater than 6 months of age with a simple febrile seizure[1].

The pathophysiology of febrile seizures is still unknown. However, it is now thought to be induced by the peak temperature, not the rate of rise of the temperature. Most families will question what their child's risk of developing epilepsy after a simple febrile seizure and whether or not their child will have recurrent seizures. It is important to counsel them that a child with a single simple febrile seizure has no increased risk when compared to general population of developing epilepsy. Approximately 1/3 of children with their first febrile seizure will experience a recurrence with 10% of these having three or more febrile seizures in a lifetime. It is very important to let the families know that the cognitive abilities of children with simple febrile seizures have been extensively studies and that they are not affected by the seizures. Table 2 outlines risk factors associated with recurrent febrile seizures and the risk of developing epilepsy.

Table 1: AAP Guidelines for Neurodiagnostic Evaluation
1. Lumbar puncture in the infant under the age of 12 months should be "strongly considered"
2. 12-18 months, careful assessment-history and physical, Lumber puncture should be "considered"
3. >18 months of age, lumbar puncture not necessary in absence of suspicious findings (nausea or vomiting)
4. Lumbar puncture with first complex febrile seizure at any age
5. Lumbar puncture if any prior antibiotic use
6. CT, MRI, EEG of limited use in initial assessment and not indicated in children with first simple febrile seizure.

Table 2: Risk Factors for Recurrent Febrile Seizures and Development of Epilepsy		
	Recurrent Febrile Seizures	**Epilepsy**
Definite Risk Factor	• Family history of febrile seizure • Age <18 months • Height of temperature • Duration of fever	• Neurodevelopmental abnormality • Complex febrile seizure • Family history of epilepsy
Possible Risk Factor	• Family history of epilepsy	• More than one complex feature
Not a Risk Factor	• Neurodevelopmental abnormality • Complex febrile seizure • More than one complex feature • Gender • Ethnicity	• Age at first febrile seizure • Height of temperature • Gender • Ethnicity

Migraine Headache

Critical Knowledge

- Common complaint in Pediatric population
- May be associated with broad neurologic symptoms

Background

Migraine headaches are relatively common in children and may mimic other disease entities, and often have broad associated symptomology. Generally onset is around 7-10 years, with girls overtaking boys in prevalence after puberty. Migraine headaches are episodic, uni or bilateral, moderate to severe in intensity and often exacerbated by activity. Frequently migraine headaches in children are associated with abdominal pain, nausea and vomiting, photo and phonophobia. Migraine headaches can also be associated with dramatic neurologic findings including stroke-like symptoms of hemiplegia, aphasia, ataxia, and visual changes. Migraines may be preceded by a neurosensory aura ("classic migraine"), frequently visual complaints. Migraine headache without aura, though, is more prevalent ("common migraine").

Multiple complex diagnostic criteria for migraine exist but in general, these include an episodic headache with three of the following

- Abdominal pain with nausea/vomiting
- Unilateral headache
- Throbbing quality
- Preceding aura
- Family history
- Relieved by sleep

Differential/Critical Concepts

The differential for headache is broad, and a careful history and exam is important to differentiate between benign and malignant causes. Generally, a diagnosis of migraine is longitudinal observation.

Although less common, consider the dangerous causes of headaches

- Any intracranial pathology
  - Mass
  - Hydrocephalus
  - Traumatic injury and intracranial hemorrhage
  - Vascular pathology
  - Idiopathic intracranial hypertension (pseudotumor cerebri)
- Tension headache
- Carbon monoxide
- Seizure

Treatment and Work-up

Children with recurrent headaches with normal neurologic findings do not routinely need neuro imaging.

Consider CT or MRI in the child with

- Dramatic change in the severity of headache
- New neurologic dysfunction
- New neurologic exam findings

(Consider ED neurology consult in the above noted conditions)

Migraine headache therapy in children can include

1. NSAIDS

2. Antiemetics
3. IV fluids
4. Dark, quiet environment

May consider

- 5-DHT agonists such as *sumitriptan*
    - Although not approved in pediatrics, safety and efficacy data supports its use
    - Consider discussing as a therapeutic option in conjunction with a neurologist
- Narcotics - be aware of rebound headache phenomena and addictive potential

Shunt Malfunction

Critical Knowledge

- Shunt malfunction may progress rapidly to coma and death
- Presenting complaint may mimic many childhood illnesses

Background

Cerebrospinal fluid shunts are frequently used in the pediatric population as a treatment for hydrocephalus. The majority are **V**etriculo **P**eritioneal (**VP**) although shunt drainage may also be vetriculopleural or ventriculoatrial, draining into the pleural space or atria respectively. It can be expected that 75% of shunts will malfunction within 10 years, with failure rates as high as 40% in the first year. Symptoms of malfunction are vague and nonspecific with headache, lethargy, vomiting and irritability being most common. A high index of suspicion must be maintained, particularly with any neurologic complaint, in the shunt patient.

Causes of Shunt Malfunction may include

- Obstruction- most frequent
- Infection
- Tubing disruption, disconnection, or migration
- Valve malfunction

Differential/Critical Concepts

- Evaluation of the shunt patient involves palpation of fluid reservoir and shunt tubing for signs of breaks, tenderness, swelling or erythema
- History should include underlying pathology and cause of hydrocephalus

- Complete neurologic exam
- Differential is broad and should include meningitis, worsening underlying disease, sepsis, otitis, gastroenteritis

Treatment and Work-up

Concern for shunt malfunction mandates

- Head CT - signs of increased or changed hydrocephalus
- Shunt series X-ray (skull, neck, chest, abdomen) - evaluate for kinks, breaks, disconnections
- Low threshold for antibiotics if fever or other signs of infection
- Neurosurgical consultation for any concern for shunt malfunction
- Shunt tap may be appropriate in consultation with neurosurgery

Questions

1. A 2 year old otherwise healthy toddler was brought in by mother after a witnessed 3 minute tonic-clonic seizure 30 minutes prior to arrival. Your exam reveals a non-toxic appearing child with a fever of 39.3, clear rhinnorhea, and an occasional cough. Your management should include
   A. ED observation and discharge with instructions on controlling fever
   B. CT head of the head, fingerstick *glucose*
   C. Admission to pediatrics to workup first time seizure
   D. Load with *phenytoin* and pediatric neurology follow up
   Answer: A
2. A 7-year old boy with a known seizure disorder is brought in by paramedics from school after a 15 minute seizure on the playground. Upon arrival to the ED, child begins with tonic/clonic activity and is unresponsive. Medics had been unsuccessful establishing IV access and no medication has been given. Initial appropriate management would include
   A. *Phenytoin* 20 mg/kg IM
   B. *Fosphenytoin* 20 mg/kg IM
   C. *Diazepam* 5 mg PO
   D. *Midazolam* 2 mg IM
   Answer: D

References

1. American Academy of Pediatrics. Provisional Committee on Quality Improvement. Practice parameter: the neurodiagnostic evaluation of the child with simple febrile seizure. *Pediatrics* 1996; 97: 769
2. Fuchs, Susan M. *Neurologic Disorders*. Pediatric Emergency Medicine. Ed. Roger M Barkin. Mosby-Year Book. 1997. 972-1024
3. Pitetti, R. Emergency Department Evaluation of Ventricular Shunt Malfunction Is the shunt series really necessary? *Pediatr Emerg Care.* 2007 Mar;23 (3):137-41
4. Kim TY, Stewart G, Voth M, Moynihan JA, Brown L. Signs and symptoms of cerebrospinal fluid shunt malfunction in the pediatric emergency department. *Pediatr Emerg Care.* 2006 Jan;22 (1):28-34
5. Lewis DW. Pediatric migraine. Pediatr Rev. 2007 Feb;28 (2):43-53.
6. De Negri M, Baglietto MG. *Treatment of status epilepticus in children.* Paediatr Drugs. 2001;3 (6):411-20.
7. Ngo, Bryan G, Holmes, James F. Performance of lumbar puncture in young children with febrile seizures. *Acad Emerg Med* 2004 11 (5) 597
8. Meyer PG, Ducrocq S, Carli P. *Pediatric neurologic emergencies.* Curr Opin Crit Care. 2001 Apr;7 (2):81-7.
9. Sogawa Y, Maytal J. Emergency department admission of children with unprovoked seizure: recurrence within 24 hours. *Pediatr Neurol.* 2006 Aug;35 (2):98-101.

Suspected Non-Accidental Trauma: Physical Abuse/Neglect

Ross Rodgers, MD
Scottsdale Emergency Associates
Scottsdale Healthcare
Scottsdale, AZ

Critical Knowledge

- Always suspect non-accidental trauma when evaluating an injured or severely ill pediatric patient
- Treat emergent injuries first
- Report all suspected cases of child abuse and neglect
- Develop a multidiscipline team for patient care and child abuse reporting
- Document and record all pertinent information
- Establish appropriate follow-up and child safety

Background and/or Epidemiology and/or Anatomy

- The four types of child abuse
    1. Physical abuse
    2. Sexual abuse
    3. Neglect
    4. Psychological abuse
- In 2004, more than 3,500,000 children were reported as abused or neglected and 872,000 were confirmed victims by child protective services resulting in over 1,400 confirmed deaths
- 38% of these confirmed deaths are a result of neglect alone
- Up to 50% of deaths resulting from abuse or neglect are not recorded making abuse and neglect the most under-recorded form of fatal maltreatment
- 76% of deaths are in victims under the age of 4
- Infant injuries are more likely closed head injury and toddler injuries more likely abdominal injuries
- The risk of pediatric death greatly increases if the initial presentation of child abuse is not recognized!

Differential Diagnosis

- Accidental closed head injury
- Accidental fractures
- Accidental soft tissue injury
- Abdominal or visceral injuries
- Osteogenesis Imperfecta
- Pediatric seizures: bleeding diatheses or coagulopathy
- Ehlers Danlos
- Dermatologic disorders (Mongolian Spots, Berloque Dermatitis, Photodermatitis, etc.)
- Ritual lesions (Cao Gio Coining, Maquas, cupping, etc.)
- Munchausen Syndrome

Critical Concepts

- Take a detailed history from those involved and interview the patient separately if time and circumstances allow.
- Pay close attention to injuries that cannot be explained by the history, a history that changes, or delay in seeking medical treatment.
- If the patient presents with obvious signs of nonaccidental trauma the history may be taken in conjunction with law enforcement and child protective services.
- A child who is lethargic, overly reserved, apneic, or convulsing should raise higher suspicion of abuse.
- The initial assessment of the pediatric patient should include a primary survey including airway, breathing and circulation and a careful examination of the patient's vital signs adjusted for age.

Closed Head Injury

- The clinical manifestations of nonaccidental head trauma can be difficult to recognize and more than 30% of cases are missed on initial presentation. Suspect this diagnosis with any change in mental status, vomiting, apnea, seizures, bradycardia, irritability, or other unexplained injuries.
- Evaluation
  - Abnormal Pediatric Glascow Coma Score (Table 1)
  - Abnormal pupil and fundoscopic exam
  - Complete neurologic exam with reflexes

- Explore lacerations
- Assess fontanel
- Palpate for asymmetry or step-offs
- Hemotypanum
- CSF otorrhea rhinorrehea
- Battle sign or raccoon eyes

- Types of intracranial bleed
  - Subdural hematoma
  - Epidural hematoma
  - Subarachnoid hemorrhage or
  - Diffuse axonal injury
- Shaken Baby Syndrome is a significant source of morbidity and mortality of infants. Approximately 25% of victims die from injuries and almost 50% have significant morbidity including neurologic, visual, motor, and cognitive impairment. The clinical findings of shaken baby are the following
  - Retinal hemorrhages
  - Intracranial trauma (particularly subdural hemorrhage)
  - Diffuse axonal injury
  - Secondary cerebral edema
  - Fractures of the posterior and anterolateral ribs

Fractures

- Approximately 30% of all pediatric fractures and 75% of fractures under the age of one are a result of inflicted injuries.
- Palpate all joints and extremities for clinical evaluation of suspected injuries.
- Any pediatric fracture can be the result of physical abuse. However, certain fractures are more likely to be associated with abuse.

Fractures Highly Associated with Abuse

- Metaphyseal including bucket handle
- Posterior rib
- Scapular
- Spinous process
- Sternal

Fractures Moderately Associated with Abuse

- Multiple fractures
- Epiphyseal
- Vertebral body or subluxation
- Digital
- Complex skull

Fractures with Low Association of Abuse

- Clavicular
- Long bone
- Linear skull

Bruises

- Bruises anywhere on the body are extremely uncommon in infants younger than 6 months. Infants who do not "cruise" rarely bruise.
- Bruising is rare in healthy children on the hands, buttocks, cheek, nose, neck, forearms, lumbar region, or chest.
- Bruising resembling the shape of an instrument or hand, "pinch mark," or linear on the buttocks are more likely nonaccidental.
- Bilateral black eyes are almost always nonaccidental unless significant trauma is involved with the injury.
- Bruises that resemble human bites should be photographed and measured for evaluation.

Burns

- Approximately 40,000 children younger than 15 years of age are hospitalized each year because of burns.
- More than 2,000 children die from burn injuries each year.
- Approximately 20% or all pediatric burns are due to abuse. Scald burns comprise 85% of all burns.
- Immersion in water at 52°C (126°F) takes 2 minutes to cause full-thickness burns compared to only 5 seconds of immersion in water at 60°C (140°F).

The Degrees or Burns

- First degree: erythema and injury only to the epidermis
- Second degree: complete epidermis with tissue loss or blisters partial thickness of dermis

- Third degree: complete dermal layer and partial subcutaneous tissue with associated structures including nerves that lead to loss of sensation. Review the pediatric burn chapter for detailed information.

The Following Burn Characteristics are more Consistent with Nonaccidental Trauma

- Involving buttocks, groin, bilateral extremities
- Sharply demarcated edges
- Stocking-glove distribution
- Full thickness
- Symmetric
- Burns neglected or older than history indicates
- Numerous lesions of varying ages
- Pattern of burn matches instrument

Neglect

- Neglect is defined as the failure of a caregiver to adequately provide safety, food, clothing, shelter, education, protection, medical/dental care, and supervision for a child.
- The evaluation of neglect is accomplished mainly though a careful history and visual observations of caregiver and patient interactions.
- Psychosocial stressors should be addressed that include poverty, unemployment, substance abuse, domestic violence, and varying discipline styles

Some Indications of Neglect

- Most clinical findings of neglect are subtle
- Failure to thrive or developmental delay
- Untreated illnesses including infections or fractures
- Lack of connection or caring in the guardian
- Physical findings such as sunken fontanel and personal hygiene appearance are the subtle nuances that should be evaluated during a pediatric examination.

Treatment

- The initial resuscitation should follow ATLS and PALS guidelines.
- Patients with head injury should receive serial neurological exams, head computed tomography, radiographic evaluation of the cervical spine, and pediatric neurosurgery consultation. The majority of pediatric intracranial bleeding is non-operative.
- Skeletal survey should be completed to evaluate for acute or chronic fractures.
- Laboratory analysis if indicated of CBC, coagulation studies, CMP, lactate, and ABG if airway compromise.
- If intra-abdominal injury is suspected prompt evaluation via ultrasound, radiography, laparoscopy, or laparotomy is needed.
- Ophthalmology consultation to evaluate for retinal hemorrhage.
- Medical or legal photography as soon as patient is stabilized.
- The key to treating non-accidental trauma is recognition!

Long Term Care Social Care

- Every State has mandated reporting laws with an established multi-disciplinary task force consisting of social work, law enforcement, child abuse specialist etc.
- Every state has standardized protocols will help ensure that all information is documented and reported correctly.
- Review state laws to determine the information that should be documented with each reported case of child abuse.
- After recognition, report to Child Protective Services or similar agency under the Child Abuse Prevention and Treatment Act.
- The agency will perform the following tasks
    - Intake of information
    - Investigation and assessment that can include a home visit
    - Case decision with voluntary or involuntary recommendations
    - Treatment and case management.
    - Placement of the child in the home, removal to foster care, or other court mandated action is based on the estimated risk of danger to the child.

- Case closure when the family has addressed all CPS needs or the child is permanently removed from the home.

Questions

1. What is the most common fracture associated with child abuse?
   A. Bucket handle fracture
   B. Linear skull fracture
   C. Long bone shaft fracture
   D. Posterior rib fracture

   Answer: D, posterior rib fractures are the most common fracture associated with child abuse.

2. Which age injury relationship is most correct?
   A. Infants more likely to present with head trauma, toddlers with abdominal trauma, and abuse related injuries decrease for school age children.
   B. Infants more likely to present with head trauma, toddlers with abdominal trauma, and abuse related injuries increase for school age children.
   C. Infants more likely to present with abdominal trauma, toddlers with head trauma, and abuse related injuries decrease for school age children.
   D. Infants more likely to present with abdominal trauma, toddlers with head trauma, and abuse related injuries increase for school age children.

   Answer: B, infants are more likely to present with head trauma, toddlers with abdominal trauma, and abuse does decrease for school age children.

3. Which of the following is true regarding child abuse reporting?
   A. All 50 states have mandated reporting laws.
   B. Failure to report suspected child abuse can result in criminal liability.
   C. The Child Abuse Prevention and Treatment Act protect any individual who reports suspected child abuse in good faith from civil or criminal liability.
   D. All of the above.

   Answer: D, all of the above statements are true.

References

1. American Academy of Pediatrics Committee on Child Abuse and Neglect: Shaken baby syndrome: inflicted cerebral trauma. *Pediatrics* 1993 Dec; 92(6): 872-5
2. American Academy of Pediatrics: *Visual Diagnosis of Child Abuse* 2nd Edition. 2003.
3. Christopher NC, Anderson D, Gaertner L, et al: Childhood injuries and the importance of documentation in the emergency department. *Pediatr Emerg Care* 1995 Feb; 11(1): 52-7
4. Council on Scientific Affairs: AMA diagnostic and treatment guidelines concerning child abuse and neglect. *JAMA* 1985 Aug 9; 254(6): 796-800
5. Crume, T., DiGuiseppi, C., Byers, T., Sirotnak, A., & Garrett, C. Underascertainment of child maltreatment fatalities by death certificates, 1990-1998. *Pediatrics, 2002; 110*(2).
6. Herman-Giddens ME, Brown G, Verbiest S, et al: Underascertainment of child abuse mortality in the United States. *JAMA* 1999 Aug 4; 282(5): 463-7
7. Hyden PW, Gallagher TA: Child abuse intervention in the emergency room. *Pediatr Clin North Am* 1992 Oct; 39(5): 1053-81
8. Kleinman PK. *Skeletal trauma: general considerations.* In: Kleinman PK, ed. Diagnostic imaging of child abuse. Baltimore: Williams & Wilkins, 1987;8-25
9. National Child Abuse and Neglect Data System: United States Health and Human Services Office of Children and Families. Website 2007 Feb: http://www.acf.hhs.gov/programs/cb/systems/index.htm
10. Sugar NF, Taylor JA, Feldman KW: *Bruises in infants and toddlers: those who don't cruise rarely bruise.* Puget Sound Pediatric Research Network. Arch Pediatr Adolesc Med 1999 Apr; 153(4): 399-403

Sexual Assault

Elizabeth Weinstein, MD
Assistant Professor of Clinical Emergency Medicine
Department of Emergency Medicine and Pediatrics
Indiana University School of Medicine
Antoinette L. Laskey, MD, MPH, FAAP
Assistant Professor of Pediatrics
Indiana University School of Medicine

Critical Knowledge

- Generally, any child with alleged assault within the preceding 72 hours requires immediate evaluation and complete exam, including genital exam and consideration for forensic evidence collection.
- Any child with alleged assault outside of the 72 hour window and without signs or symptoms of acute injury, infection or pregnancy, or compelling reason to believe there may be recoverable forensic evidence, may have the genital exam deferred to a child advocacy specialist (Child Abuse Pediatrics) at a later date; but, they should have a full medical screening exam. Appropriate authorities should be notified and the child's safety and safety of other potentially at risk children must be ensured.
- The interview should be conducted by someone trained in forensic interviewing, and whenever possible deferred to an advocacy center or similar facility. Physician interview of the patient should include pertinent medical history only, as the physician may otherwise inadvertently contaminate the historical evidence and damage any legal case.
- Virginity CANNOT be determined from an exam.
- Prepubertal children SHOULD NOT undergo speculum exam. Post-pubertal girls do not necessarily require speculum exam.
- Children should NOT undergo forced genital exam, *unless,* there is concern for significant injury. (i.e., forensic evidence collection alone does not warrant an exam under anesthesia.) When there is concern for significant injury exam under anesthesia may be appropriate.
- *Most* pediatric victims of sexual assault have NORMAL exams.
- Penetration to adults means penetration of the vaginal orifice or anus. Children often interpret penetration as penetration of the labia or buttocks.
- Highly suspicious injuries include transections of the posterior hymen (from 3 to 9 o'clock in the dorsal lithotomy or frog leg position) bruising

or bleeding of the posterior fourchette, acute laceration or bruising of the hymen, vaginal lacerations, deep perianal lacerations, bruising of the penis.[1]

- Infection with chlamydia, gonorrhea, or syphilis in a prepubertal child outside of the perinatal period is considered diagnostic of sexual contact, and depending on the age of the child, sexual abuse.

Definition

"*Sexual abuse occurs when a child is engaged in sexual activities that he or she cannot comprehend, for which he or she is developmentally unprepared and cannot give consent, and/or which violate the law or social taboos of society. [These] may include all forms of oral-genital, genital, or anal contact by or to the child or abuse that does not involve contact, such as exhibitionism, voyeurism, or using the child in the production of pornography.*"[2]

Epidemiology

- 12-25% of girls and 8-10% of boys in the US have been victims of sexual assault by the age of 18.[2]
- Children less than 18 years of age comprise 2/3 of all victims of sexual abuse reported to law enforcement in the US, 1/3 are under age 12.[3]
- Adolescents comprise the largest group of victims.[4] Most know their perpetrator.

Anatomy

(Diagram of female genitals – labia minora and majora, clitoris, urethra, vagina, hymen, posterior fourchette, fossa navicularis, perineal body, anus)

(Diagram of male genitals - glans, shaft, anus, perineum, scrotum)

The Chief Complaint

- Reasons for referral for exam for suspected abuse: the child has made a disclosure; the child has exhibited a change in behavior; the child has been noted to have an abnormal physical exam; the child has been exposed to an abuse situation or possible abuse situation.
- Behavioral changes that may prompt referral include: sexualized behavior or knowledge inappropriate for age, masturbation that is beyond normal developmental expectations, new onset enuresis/encopresis, sleep/appetite disturbances, and other behavioral changes such as declining school performance or aggression.

The History

- *Medical history* should be obtained by the physician to include: menstrual history (including tampon use and frequency/length of cycle), surgeries and previous illnesses/chronic illnesses; thorough review of systems including GI, GU (including history of enuresis, encopresis, hematuria, or hematochezia), hematology and dermatology. Time of last shower/bath, last urination/defecation or brushing of teeth should be obtained if evidence collection is going to be attempted. Any changes in sleeping, eating or school performance should also be documented.
- *Sexual history* is NOT indicated
- *Family history* should be obtained
- *History of the allegation/events* and thorough *social history* may be obtained from the accompanying adult with the child absent for this portion of the interview. History should include who lives in the home, other adult contacts, history of previous sexual maltreatment, and other previous contacts with Child Protective Services or Law Enforcement.
- Improper questioning of children can have catastrophic results for legal proceedings. Consequently, history of events/allegations by the child should be obtained by a specialist trained to perform pediatric forensic interviews – often at child advocacy centers or by law enforcement.[5] Any spontaneous disclosures made by the child should be documented verbatim with the use of quotation marks.

The Exam

Timing & Location

- In general, immediate exam is indicated if the alleged event occurred within the preceding 72 hours or if there is concern for injury. The exam should include forensic evidence collection and a complete medical screening exam.
- Any child with alleged assault outside of the 72 hour window and without signs or symptoms of acute injury, infection or pregnancy, or compelling reason to believe there may be recoverable forensic evidence, may have the genital exam deferred to a child advocacy specialist at a later date; but, they should have a full medical screening exam. Appropriate authorities should be notified and the child's safety and safety of other potentially at risk children must be ensured.

Preparing the for the Exam

- Explain the exam to the patient beforehand.
- The child should be allowed to have a trusted adult accompany him or her in the exam room if the child chooses.
- At a minimum, one additional medical personnel should be in the exam room with the examiner. This provides a chaperone and helps facilitate the exam and evidence collection.

Step-by-Step Exam

- Begin with general and non-threatening exam components that are more familiar to children (listening to the heart and lungs, looking in the ears and mouth, etc.) and progress to the genital exam as the child becomes more comfortable.
- Perform a comprehensive exam for any indications of physical abuse. Evaluate the child's skin and document any bruising. Be specific about size and location. Do NOT estimate age of bruising or other trauma. Evaluate the oropharynx with particular attention to any palatal petechia or tears of the labial or lingular frenula. Evaluate the medial thighs for any injury or bruising. All bruises, bite-marks, or other lesions should be photographed with a ruler included in the frame for reference.
- Positioning the child for ano-genital exam: Position of choice is child dependent. Younger children are generally examined in a supine frog leg position on an exam table or in a caregiver's lap. Adolescents may prefer a stirrup position. Boys can have an adequate exam in the lateral recumbent position which may be less stressful than knee chest. However, on occasion, further evaluation of possible injury is best performed in the knee chest position.
- Visualization of the hymen, vestibule and vaginal opening is achieved by applying gentle outward labial traction to the labia majora; in pubertal patients, a cotton swab *moistened* with *preservative-free saline* can be used to help fully visualize the hymen when hymenal folds are present.
- In prepubertal children the hymen is very sensitive and touching it can be painful for the patient. In these patients manipulating the labial traction can often provide adequate views.
- Photo documentation of the ano-genital exam with colposcopy should be obtained whenever possible.
- Digital Rectal exam is not indicated.[5]

- Document Tanner staging. (see accompanying chart)
- If swabs are indicated, care should be taken to insert the cotton swab into the vaginal canal without touching the hymenal walls. Cervical swabs are unnecessary in prepubertal children and may not be necessary in the adolescent patient. A genital wash may also be employed. Fill syringe with *saline* and wash the perineum catching the run-off on a 2x2.

Forensic Evidence Collection

General Rules

- Follow guidelines of your specific evidence collection kit as these can vary.
- Urine should be collected AFTER the genital exam so as not to eliminate possible forensic evidence.
- Maintain chain of evidence: seal, label and initial all samples; date and time everything, including times of transfer of custody; document agency and name of individual accepting forensic evidence for police custody.[6]
- Avoid transfer of trace evidence: separate all collected items; change gloves when changing sites of collection.[6]
- Protect integrity of samples: Do not heat dry samples. Air dry only; refrigerate any blood and body fluid samples; use only paper and glass. Do not use plastic.[6]

What to Collect

- UPT should be obtained, even in the absence of reported onset of menarche, if the child is Tanner stage appropriate
- History, timing, nature of contact and sex of perpetrator help to determine if a child needs to be swabbed for forensic evidence.[1] In general children should be swabbed if there has been genital-genital contact, oral-genital contact, and/or anal-genital contact or if there is a history of ejaculation.
- Black light (Wood's lamp) should be used to evaluate for other areas to swab for secretions.
- Collect the child's clothing or bedding as forensic evidence is frequently collected from these sources.[1]
- Scrape underneath the child's fingernails if there appears to be any material or if there is any report of the child scratching the alleged perpetrator.
- Comb pubic hair, if present, and there is report of genital contact.
- Use floss sticks to collect evidence that may be trapped between teeth in cases of oral genital contact.

Testing for STDs

- Approximately 5% of abused children acquire an STD. Numbers are higher in the adolescent population, but STDs do occur in prepubertal abuse as well.[7,2]
- Testing in prepubertal children should be obtained if: the child is symptomatic (e.g., discharge, dysuria), the perpetrator is known to have an STD or risk factors for STD, there is history of genital-to-genital contact, or there is genital injury.[8]
- In prepubertal children, infection with chlamydia, gonorrhea, or syphilis outside of the perinatal period is considered diagnostic of abuse. Infection with HIV without other identified risk factors is similarly considered diagnostic. Trichomonas vaginalis infection is considered highly suspicious. Condylomata acuminate and genital herpes are considered suspicious.[8]
- Adolescent victims should be tested for STDs.[9]
- Adolescents who have been raped should have serum samples testing for HIV, syphilis and HBV (to demonstrate lack or presence of preexisting infection.) HBV and syphilis testing needs to be repeated at 6 weeks, HIV at 3-6 months.[8,9]
- If STD testing is indicated vaginal/urethral swabs should be sent for *C trachomatis* and *N gonorrhea* culture (PCR is inadequate to establish legal proof of infection in prepubertal children. In adolescents PCR *may* be sufficient as long as there is a confirmatory test of a different part of the genome). (Meatal specimen discharge in place of intra-urethral swab is considered adequate in boys.) Vaginal swabs should be sent for culture for *trichomonas vaginalis* and wet mount. If history indicates oral-genital or anal-genital contact, swabs from the oropharynx and anus should also be obtained.[2]
- Any lesions suspicious for herpes should be cultured for HSV 1 & 2.
- Testing for HIV, hepatitis B &C and syphilis may vary depending on exposure, age of the child, knowledge of the perpetrator's risk factors, local prevalence, and family wishes.
- Prophylactic/empiric therapy should NOT be instituted unless cultures have been obtained and is generally not recommended for asymptomatic prepubertal children.[6,8]

Differential Diagnosis: Findings Confused with Sexual Abuse

- Traumatic: straddle injuries (there should be NO injury to the hymen as this is a very internal structure, but there may be labial bruising)[6], toilet lid injuries to penis, self inflicted injuries
- Dermatologic: lichen sclerosis, henoch-schönlein purpura
- Non-specific vaginitis: irritant (bubble-bath, soaps, fecal contamination, etc.)
- Infectious vaginitis: *staphylococcus aureus,* group A streptococcus, candida, etc.
- Urinary tract infections
- Anal fissures
- Pre-pubertal vaginal bleeding: arteriovenous malformations, foreign body, hormonal glitches, urethral prolapse
- Peri-anal group A streptococcal infections

Myth Busting

- Virginity CANNOT be determined from physical exam.
- The size of the hymenal opening changes with relaxation and position, it does NOT prove penetration.
- In the vast majority of established cases of sexual abuse, even those in which penetration has taken place, the examination is NORMAL.[10,12]

Treatment

Chlamydia/GC/Trich

- Prophylaxis for GC/chlamydia and trichomonas should be provided for adolescent assault victims.[8]
- Prophylaxis for asymptomatic pre-pubertal children is not generally recommended, though may instituted because of familial wishes or other concerns.[6,8]

Selected Treatment Options[13]

	Weight <45 kg	Weight >45 kg
Gonorrhea	*Ceftriaxone* 125 mg IM, single dose	*Ceftriaxone* 125 mg IM, single dose
alternative therapy	------------------	*Cefixime* 400 mg PO, single dose

Selected Treatment Options[13]		
	Weight <45 kg	**Weight >45 kg**
Chlamydia Trachomatis	*Azithromycin* 20 mg/kg (maximum 1 gm) PO, single dose	*Azithromycin* 1 gm PO, single dose
alternative therapy	*Erythromycin* base 50 mg/kg/day divided qid for 14 days duration	*Doxycycline* 100 mg PO BID for 7 days duration (must be at least 8 years old)
Trichomoniasis & Bacterial Vaginosis	*Metronidazole* 15 mg/kg/day PO divided tid for 7 days duration	*Metronidazole* 2 g PO, single dose

HIV

- HIV infection has been reported in children with sexual abuse as the only established risk factor.[8,9]
- Efficacy of post exposure prophylaxis in the setting of sexual assault is theoretical and based on reduction of transmission of HIV in occupational exposures and in the reduction of vertical transmission from HIV positive mothers to the fetus[8,14]
- Prophylaxis may be indicated depending on risk assessment.
- Risk assessment: receptive anal intercourse and receptive vaginal intercourse carry the highest risk for infection. Risk is elevated in the presence of mucosal injury. Risk assessment should include HIV serostatus of the perpetrator if known, or risk factors of the perpetrator (IVDA, incarceration history, etc.) if known. Number of assailants and history of ejaculation should also be considered.[8,14]
- Compliance with medication continuation and follow-up is very poor. A frank discussion with the family regarding risk-benefit and drug toxicities should take place before therapy is initiated.[14]
- There are no evidence-based guidelines for initiation of therapy and drug regimen in this population; however, if the child presents within the initial 72 hours following potential exposure baseline HIV testing in the ED and initiation of a 4 week course of 2 drug therapy (generally *zidovudine* and *lamivudine*) may be employed.[14,15] In very high risk situations, a third agent, generally a protease inhibitor may be added. Side effects dramatically increase with the addition of a third agent.

- Two drug therapy cost is approximately $1,000 for a one month supply and may or may not be covered by insurance.[14]
- If treatment is being considered, consultation with a specialist in treating HIV in children is recommended.[8] Baseline complete blood count and blood chemistries including transaminases should also be obtained.
- If treatment is initiated the family should be provided with sufficient medication to last until follow up within 3-7 days. At that time the child should be reassessed for side-effects and tolerance.
- National Clinician's Post Exposure Hotline (PEPLine): 888-448-4911.

Hepatitis B

HBV vaccination is recommended for those with an incomplete vaccination series and for those who have negative surface antibodies (however, serologies may not be ordered in cases in which the contact would not warrant concern of transmission (e.g., fondling)[8]

Pregnancy Prevention

Emergency contraception should be offered in assaults that could potentially result in pregnancy.[9]

Follow-up

- Children reporting sexual assault need to be believed, protected and supported: treatment should include follow-up with a primary care physician as soon as is reasonable following the event and referral for counseling/ support services.
- For STD concerns, in children who do not receive empiric therapy, additional follow up for reexamination should be arranged for 2 weeks and 12 weeks.[8] For adolescents, follow-up for STD check should occur in 1-2 weeks.
- Any child with injury should have urgent follow-up to ensure that the injury is healing properly. This may be with a Child Abuse Specialist or with the child's primary care physician.

Legal Issues

Mandatory Reporting

- All 50 states have mandatory reporting laws that include medical personnel. These laws protect the reporter from civil litigation in good faith reports. Failure to report, in cases in which there is concern, has resulted in law suits. Any child with complaint of assault or concern for maltreatment or neglect must be reported. Reporting requirements for sexual activity between consenting minors varies from state to state. You should be aware of your state's individual reporting requirements.

- HIPAA does not trump mandated reporting laws.
- HIPAA does allow for the release of information related to child abuse and neglect of ongoing criminal investigations. However, you MUST document who you are disclosing information to.

Documentation

- Document what questions were asked and what answers were given and by whom. Try to use direct, complete quotes whenever possible and use quotation marks when charting.
- Draw specific diagrams, including location and sizes of all lesions.
- Document chain of evidence information as previously detailed.

Working with Child Protective Services

- Once Child Protective Services (CPS) has been involved, clarify what conditions need to be met before the child can be released from the hospital and to whom the child may be released.
- Guidelines may vary by state or jurisdiction. Generally, social work can you help you determine the guidelines where you practice.

Resources

1. National Children's Alliance: www.nca-online.org
2. Regional Children's Advocacy Centers
3. Midwest Regional Children's Advocacy Center
   www.mrcac.org
   (888) 422-2955
   (651) 220-6750
4. Southern Regional Children's Advocacy Center
   www.nationalcac.org/professionals/srcac
   (800) 747-8122
   (704) 285-9588
5. Northeast Regional Children's Advocacy Center
   www.nrcac.org
   (800) 662-4124
6. Western Regional Children's Advocacy Center
   (800) 582-2203

Recommended Additional References

- Kellogg, N. and N. American Academy of Pediatrics Committee on Child Abuse and, *The evaluation of sexual abuse in children.* Pediatrics, 2005. 116(2): p. 506-12.
- Bernard, D., P. Melissa, and K. Makoroff, *The Evaluation of Suspected Pediatric Sexual Abuse.* Clinical Pediatric Emergency Medicine, 2006. 7(3): p. 9.
- American College of Emergency Physicians, *Evaluation and Management of the Sexually Assaulted or Sexually Abused Patient.* 1999, Dallas: American College of Emergency Physicians.
- Center for Disease Control and Prevention. *Sexually Transmitted Diseases Treatment Guidelines 2006: Sexual Assault and STDs.* 2006 Available from: http://www.cdc.gov/std/treatment/2006/sexual-assault.htm.

Normal Hymenal Patterns

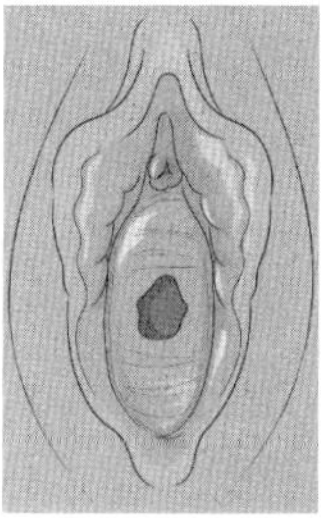

Annular

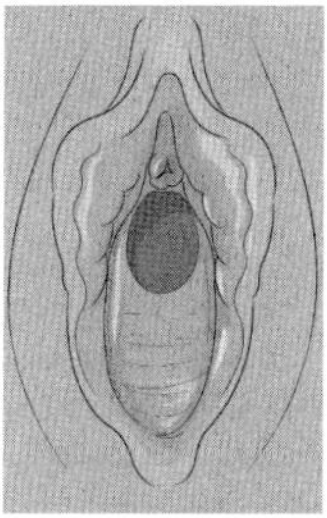

Crescentic

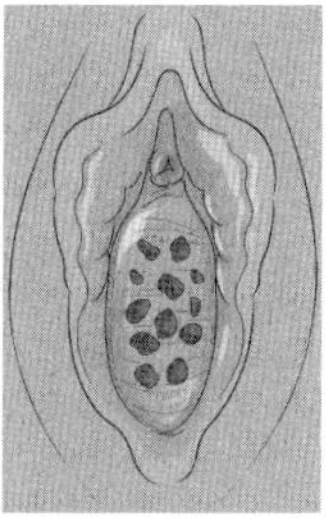

Cribriform

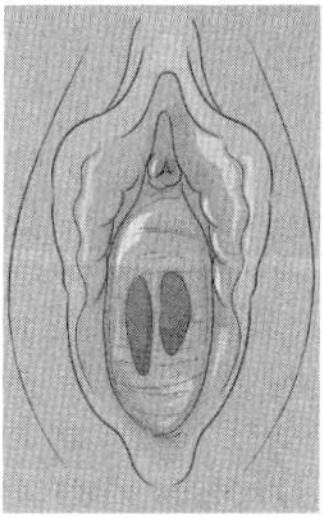

Septate

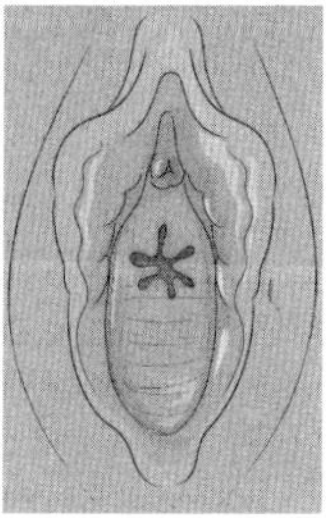

Redundant

Tanner Stage	Female Breast	Male Penis/ Scrotum	Pubic Hair
1	Prepubertal. No glandular tissue.	Prepubertal (testicular volume less than 1.5 ml; small penis)	None
2	Breast bud forms, with small area of surrounding glandular tissue; areola begins to widen	Penile length unchanged. testicular volume increases (1.6 and 6 ml) skin on scrotum thins, reddens and enlarges	Scant long, downy, slightly pigmented hair at the base of the penis and scrotum or on the labia majora
3	Breast becomes more elevated, and extends beyond the borders of the areola. Areola further widens.	Penis lengthens. Scrotum further enlarges. Testicular volume (6-12 ml)	Hair becomes more course and curly and extends laterally
4	Further increased breast size and elevation; areola and papilla form a secondary mound projecting from the contour of the surrounding breast	Penis increases in length and circumference. Scrotum enlarges and darkens. Testicular volume 12-20 ml.	Adult like hair but spares medial thigh
5	Adult pattern. Areola returns to contour of the surrounding breast.	Adult Pattern	Adult pattern

Questions

1. The following testing is appropriate in an 9 year-old child complaining of vaginal discharge and sexual assault
   A. Vaginal swab for GC/chlamydia PCR and trichomonas; serum for hepatitis B & C
   B. Cervical swab for GC/chlamydia culture and trichomonas; serum for hepatitis B & C
   C. Cervical swab for GC/chlamydia PCR and trichomonas; serum for hepatitis B & C
   D. Vaginal swab for GC/chlamydia culture and trichomonas; serum for hepatitis B & C

   Answer: D. PCR is inadequate to establish legal proof of infection in prepubertal children. Culture is required. Vaginal exam is sufficient. Cervical exam is not indicated.

2. A child presents to the emergency department after disclosing to her teacher that she has been touched inappropriately by her mother's boyfriend on several occasions. The last assault was over 92 hours ago. Which of the following is not true?
   A. You should avoid questioning the child about her disclosure and defer this aspect of the history to someone trained in forensic interviewing
   B. Genital exam can almost always be deferred to a child protection specialist if alleged assault occurred more than 72 prior.
   C. If the child refuses a speculum exam, it is appropriate to perform an exam under anesthesia for evidence collection.
   D. Child Protective Services must be notified and the child's safety assured prior to release.

   Answer: C. The only indication for exam under anesthesia is concern for significant injury that requires visualization and intervention. When at all possible history and questions about the disclosure should be deferred to a specialist trained in forensic interviewing so as to avoid possibly contaminating the history. Child protective services must be notified and the child's safety ensured prior to discharge.

3. Which of the following statements regarding reporting is NOT true?
   A. A physician is a mandated reporter. Failure to report may be actionable.
   B. HIPAA prevents physicians from sharing information regarding child abuse to law enforcement without guardian consent.
   C. You may be sued by a party for reporting suspected abuse if the party is subsequently found to be innocent of any wrong doing.

   Answer: C. Reporters are protected from suite after good faith reporting. There have been successful legal cases against physicians for failing to recognize and/or report suspected abuse.

References

1. Palusci, V.J., et al., *Urgent medical assessment after child sexual abuse.* Child Abuse & Neglect, 2006. 30(4): p. 367-80.
2. Kellogg, N. and N. American Academy of Pediatrics Committee on Child Abuse and, The evaluation of sexual abuse in children. *Pediatrics*, 2005. 116(2): p. 506-12.

3. Howard N. Snyder, P.D., *Sexual Assault of Young Children as Reported to Law Enforcement: Victim, Incident, and Offender Characteristics*. 2000, U.S Department of Justice, Bureau of Justice Statistics. p. ii-14.
4. Young, K.L., et al., *Forensic laboratory evidence in sexually abused children and adolescents*. Archives of Pediatrics & Adolescent Medicine, 2006. 160(6): p. 585-8.
5. Bernard, D., P. Melissa, and K. Makoroff, *The Evaluation of Suspected Pediatric Sexual Abuse*. Clinical Pediatric Emergency Medicine, 2006. 7(3): p. 9.
6. Physicians, A.C.o.E., *Evaluation and Management of the Sexually Assaulted or Sexually Abused Patient*. 1999, Dallas: American College of Emergency Physicians.
7. Siegel RM, S.C.e.a., The prevalence of sexually transmitted diseases in children and adolescents evaluated for sexual abuse in Cincinnati: rationale for limited STD testing in prepubertal girls. *Pediatrics*, 1995. 96(6): p. 5.
8. CDC. *Sexually Transmitted Diseases Treatment Guidelines 2006: Sexual Assault and STDs*. 2006 [cited; Available from: http://www.cdc.gov/std/treatment/2006/sexual-assault.htm.
9. Kaplan, D.W., et al., Care of the adolescent sexual assault victim. *Pediatrics*, 2001. 107(6): p. 1476-9.
10. Heger, A., et al., *Children referred for possible sexual abuse: medical findings in 2384 children*. Child Abuse & Neglect, 2002. 26(6-7): p. 645-59.
11. Adams, J.A., et al., Examination findings in legally confirmed child sexual abuse: it's normal to be normal.[see comment]. *Pediatrics*, 1994. 94(3): p. 310-7.
12. Kellogg, N., S.W. Menard, and A. Santos, Genital Anatomy in Pregnant Adolescents: "Normal" Does Not Mean "Nothing Happened." *Pediatrics*, 2004. 113(1): p. 3.
13. Pickering LK, B.C., Long SS, McMillan JA, eds., *Red Book: 2006 Report of the Committee on Infectious Diseases* 27th ed. 2006, Elk Grove Village: American Academy of Pediatrics. 992.
14. Schremmer, R.D., D. Swanson, and K. Kraly, *Human immunodeficiency virus postexposure prophylaxis in child and adolescent victims of sexual assault*. Pediatric Emergency Care, 2005. 21(8): p. 502-6.
15. Babl, F.E., et al., *Prophylaxis against possible human immunodeficiency virus exposure after nonoccupational needlestick injuries or sexual assaults in children and adolescents*. Archives of Pediatrics & Adolescent Medicine, 2001. 155(6): p. 680-2.

The Normal Newborn Examination

Merlin C. Lowe, MD
Department of Pediatrics
The University of Arizona

Critical Knowledge

- A newborn examination in the emergency room should be quick yet thorough. A systematic approach to the exam will ensure nothing is missed.
- A thorough physical examination can help determine how best to proceed with evaluation of the infant.
- Recognizing age appropriate variations in the examination, especially regarding vital signs, can be difficult. Using a quick reference card can help provide easy recall.
- Recognizing common anatomical variations in the newborn examination can prevent an unnecessary work-up.

Background

Newborns will present to the emergency room for many reasons. A quick, yet thorough examination will allow the provider to proceed with the work up of the infant in an organized, effective fashion. Some infants will be brought to the emergency room when they are well; some will be brought to the emergency room with true illnesses. Being able to distinguish between a normal and abnormal neonatal exam can provide clues to guide further evaluation.

Epidemiology

Minor anomalies will be found in 15-20% of newborns. These infants have a 3% chance of having a major anomaly. When the number of minor anomalies rises to two or three the risk of a major anomaly rises to 10 and 20 percent, respectively.

Infant Vital Signs

Age	Heart Rate	Respiratory Rate	Systolic Blood Pressure
Newborn	90-180	40-60	60-90
1 month	110-180	30-50	70-104
3 months	110-180	30-45	70-104
6 months	110-180	20-35	72-110

1 year	80-170	20-30	72-115

- Temperature is a crucial part of the vital sign evaluation. One should be aware of high temperatures as well as low temperatures as both can be indicators of infection. Keep in mind that infection is not the only cause of temperature fluctuation. Hypothermia may be a sign of hypoglycemia, hypothyroidism or hypoxia. Hyperthermia may also represent adrenal hemorrhage, intracranial hemorrhage, or drug withdrawal.
- Knowing appropriate vital signs for age is crucial to the accurate ability of the clinician to recognize potential problems.
- It is recommended that a quick reference chart for pediatric vital signs be kept available for review.

General Evaluation

- One of the clinician's greatest tools to evaluate a newborn is the general impression one gets of an infant.
- Does the infant appear vigorous and alert or ill and toxic?
- Look for signs of distress including labored breathing, persistent crying and irritability with difficulty consoling the infant.
- A non-vigorous infant should be a red flag to seek for an underlying issue.

Evaluation of the Head

- The anterior fontanel can remain open until approx. age 18 months although it often is quite small by age 12 months. An enlarged anterior fontanel can be an indication of hypothyroidism.
- The posterior fontanel is generally fully closed by age 12 months.
- The fontanelles should be examined to ensure that they are soft and flat.
  - A bulging fontanel is an indicator of increased intracranial pressure.
  - A sunken fontanel may indicate dehydration.
- Significant molding can follow a vaginal birth. This generally resolves in three to five days.
- One should also examine for any evidence of a caput succedaneum or hemorrhages (such as a cephalhematoma) related to birth trauma. (see Figure next page) Extraction deliveries increase the risk of developing such a bleed.
- Suture lines should be examined for evidence of excessive widening as an indicator of increased intracranial pressure, possibly from an underlying hydrocephalus.

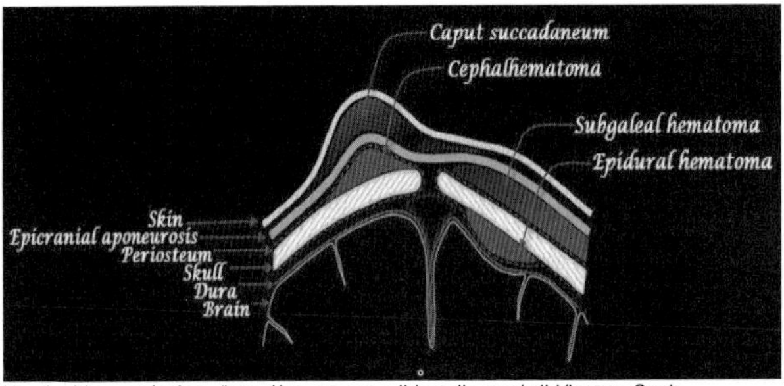

Used with permission. (http://commons.wikimedia.org/wiki/Image:Scalp_hematomas.jpg)

Eyes

- Red reflexes are assessed by viewing the pupil through the ophthalmoscope at least a few inches back from the eye. One should note color and symmetry of the red reflexes bilaterally.
  - A white reflex (leukocoria) may be indicative of several processes including retinoblastoma, glaucoma, cataracts, or vitreous opacities.
  - A finding of leukocoria requires evaluation by an ophthalmologist.
- Extra-ocular movements should also be examined. Dysconjugate gaze at birth is not particularly concerning. This finding should resolve by two months of age. Persistent dysconjugate gaze should be evaluated.
- Subconjunctival hemorrhages are quite common following birth and are not dangerous. They typically will resolve within 1-2 weeks.

Ears

- Ear positioning should be evaluated. Low set ears have been associated with several genetic syndromes.
- Pre-auricular skin tags or pits are quite common and often will run in families. Previously it was thought they were associated with other anomalies; however, further testing has shown that they are generally inconsequential and do not require further workup.
- Ear anomalies (such as malformed auricles) can be associated with other anomalies, in particular anomalies of the genitourinary tract. A renal ultrasound is generally recommended in these patients.

Mouth

- The mouth should be examined for any oral lesions. A finger can be inserted into the mouth to check for a cleft palate.
- About 1 in 3,000 infants will have a natal tooth. These need not be removed unless they pose a risk for aspiration or if they prevent proper feeding. If not removed, these teeth often fall out without difficulty.
- Epstein's Pearls or Bohn Nodules may be seen in the mouth of an infant as well. These are yellowish or white and slightly raised nodules located near the midpalatal raphe at the junction of the hard and soft palates. These resolve spontaneously.

Neck

- Congenital muscular torticollis has an incidence of 1 in 250 live births and is known to be more common in breech and forceps deliveries. It presents with the infant keeping the head flexed and turned with the chin towards to unaffected side. 2/3rd of cases will have a palpable mass within the involved sternocleidomastoid muscle.
- Thyroglossal duct cysts may present as a midline neck mass.
- Branchial cleft anomalies can present as cysts, sinuses or pits along the ear, preauricular space and lateral neck.

Chest/Lungs

- When examining the chest, one must remember to examine all structures of the chest, including bones, lungs, and heart.
- Clavicle fractures following birth have an incidence of 0.2-3.5%. Crepitus can be felt when palpating the fractured clavicle. X-ray can confirm its presence if needed. No specific treatment is needed since they heal quite well, including severely angulated fractures.
- The lung exam should start by visualization of the infant breathing and looking for nasal flaring, grunting, retractions, symmetrical chest rise, etc.
- Transient tachypnea of the newborn will often follow cesarean section births but can be seen with vaginal births as well. Infants may need some ventilatory support; however, full recovery is expected within 24 to 72 hours.
- Fever and tachypnea is very concerning for pneumonia. In the absence of tachypnea pneumonia is unlikely in pediatric patients.

Cardiovascular

- At birth, a complex series of events must occur for the neonatal circulatory system to function properly.
  - The foramen ovale must close
  - The ductus arteriosus must close
  - Pulmonary pressures must drop
- The ductus arteriosus functionally closes around 10 to 15 hours after birth. It permanently fuses closed by approx. 3 weeks. In infants with ductal dependant lesions, the PDA may remain open longer causing their presentation to be outside this 5 hour window. (It would not be uncommon for the duct to remain open for nearly a week in some cases.)
- Due to increased pulmonary pressures, S2 may not be split. As pressures decrease to baseline, S2 will become more physiologically split. An S3 may be heard near the apex and is considered normal. An S4 is never normal in a newborn.
- The cardiac exam in a newborn relies very much on information beyond the auscultation of the heart. Palpation of peripheral pulses can detect coarctation of the aorta, for example.
- Newborns can present with several murmurs. Distinguishing between innocent murmurs and pathological ones can be difficult. When uncertain, it is always best to request a cardiology evaluation and echocardiogram.
- Innocent murmurs are quite common at birth. They typically are heard best at the left lower sternal border and have a vibratory sound to them. They typically do not radiate and are graded as I-II/VI in nature. Innocent murmurs include venous hums, pulmonary ejection murmurs, peripheral pulmonic stenosis, and Still's murmurs.
- Harsh sounding murmurs should not be attributed to innocent murmurs, nor should holosystolic or diastolic murmurs.
- Ventricular septal defects are the most common cause of a holosystolic murmur. Other possibilities include mitral or tricuspid regurgitation or other variations of VSD's such as atrioventricular septal defects.
- Some syndromes are more commonly associated with heart defects. For example, approximately 30% of those with an AVSD will be found to have Down Syndrome.

Abdomen

- Assessment should include examination for hepatomegaly, splenomegaly, and enlarged kidneys. The umbilical cord should also be inspected in newly born infants.
- The liver edge of a newborn will often be palpable approx. 1 centimeter below the costal margin. This is considered acceptable for neonates. Tables exist for appropriate liver spans in neonates and should be referenced when a question exists. In general, a liver span greater than 3.5 cm below the costal margin is considered enlarged.
- A spleen should generally not be palpable. A palpable spleen in the setting of jaundice should make one consider a hemolyzing state such as cell type incompatibility (ABO or Rh, for example) or defect in red cell morphology (spherocytosis, etc.)
- One should also remember that lung hyperinflation can move the liver and spleen downward leading to an exam consistent with hepatosplenomegaly but liver and spleen spans will be normal.
- 0.2-1% of infants will have a single umbilical artery (2 vessel cord). These infants have an increased incidence of severe renal anomalies and renal malformation (3 fold and 6 fold, respectively) over the general population.
- A scaphoid abdomen in a newly delivered infant should alert the physician to the possibility of a congenital diaphragmatic hernia. CDH is an indication for immediate intubation following delivery to minimize chances of air inflating the stomach and further compressing thoracic structures. Bag-valve mask ventilation is contraindicated with CDH.

Genitourinary Tract

- Boys should be examined for inguinal hernias, varicoceles, hydroceles, normal testes, and urethral anomalies (such as hypospadias).
- Inguinal hernias present as a bulge in the inguinal area or in the scrotum. If a hernia is detected, light, constant pressure should be applied to attempt to reduce the hernia.
- Girls can present with inguinal hernias as well, although the male to female ratio is 6:1. Presentation is as a bulge in the inguinal area.
- Varicoceles develop from a dilation of the pampiniform plexus and internal spermatic vein. They are more common on the left and more easily seen with the patient in an upright position.
- Hydroceles form from a failure of the processus vaginalis to fully close

allowing fluid, but not bowel, into the scrotum. Transillumination of the scrotum will allow differentiation of a hydrocele from a varicocele. Hydroceles transilluminate nicely while varicoceles do not.

- Ambiguous genitalia can result from girls that are virilized or boys that are undermasculinized. Phenotypes can be nearly normal female to nearly normal male or anywhere in between.
  - Boys present with ambiguous genitalia due to defective androgen synthesis or end-organ resistance to androgens.
  - Girls most commonly present with ambiguous genitalia due to congenital adrenal hyperplasia (most commonly due to 21-hydroxylase deficiency).
- Examination for ambiguous genitalia should include evaluation for clitoromegaly, micropenis, fused labia or bifid scrotum.

Extremities

- Examination should include evaluation for polydactyly, most commonly involving the "pinky" finger. Extra digits may range from a skin tag to fully formed phalanges. Toes may also be involved.
- A unilateral single, transverse palmar crease is found in approx. 4% of the general population. 1% will have a bilateral single crease. Single creases are associated with several syndromes so, when present, other anomalies should be evaluated for on physical exam.
- Unilateral club foot is found in 1 in 1,000 live births. Bilateral club feet are found in 30 to 50% of cases. Treatment is initially with serial casting. If this fails, surgery may be needed.

Neurological

- Time may not permit a full neurological exam but a general assessment of neurological status should be done on all infants, with emphasis on tone, primitive reflexes, and a gross evaluation of cranial nerves as well as muscular and sensory status.
- One should assess for symmetric facies and movement of all extremities. The infant should react to stimuli (light touch and pinprick).
- Hypotonia is an important finding to note as it is the most common neurological sign seen in infants and is associated with various syndromes.
- One should also assess whether or not the infant is meeting developmental milestones.
- Focal deficits may be an indication of plexus palsy.

Primitive Reflexes (limited listing)

Rooting reflex	Touch newborn's cheek and infant turns toward side touched.
Walking reflex	With baby upright, baby will make walking movements when foot touched to ground.
Tonic neck reflex (Fencing reflex)	Turn baby's head to one side. The chin side arm will extend and the occiput side arm will flex above the shoulder.
Moro reflex	Baby will extend then contract arms and grimaces when baby is gently released to fall a few inches.
Palmar reflex	Stroking or lightly pressing the palm/sole causes the fingers/toes to curl.
Babinski reflex	Stroking the outer edge of the sole causes the toes to spread and the great toe to dorsiflex.

Skin

- Several common neonatal skin conditions should be recognized in order to prevent an extensive, unnecessary evaluation of the infant for pathology.
- Erythema toxicum will effect up to 50% of full term infants. It typically presents within the first 2-3 days of life and resolves within a week. Lesions have a central papule surrounded by an erythematous base.
- Pustular melanosis affects approx. 5% of black infants and less than 1% of white infants. The pustules are present at birth or develop within 24 hours. The pustules subsequently rupture leaving a classic collarette of skin with hyperpigmentation of the area. At birth, the pustules may have all ruptured leaving only the collarettes.
- Milia are classically found on the nose but may also be seen on other parts of the body. They are small cysts filled with keratinocytes and skin debris.
- Neonatal acne typically will develop between the 2nd and 4th week of life. It peaks in intensity around 8-12 weeks and subsequently resolves. Typically, intervention is not needed; however, some cases may progress to severe nodulocystic acne. In these cases, medical management can help prevent scarring.
- Angel kisses and stork bites (seen on the eyelids and nape of the neck, respectively) represent nevi simplex. These will typically fade with increasing age, though some will remain.
- Nevus flamus, or port-wine stain, often will be more extensive than a nevus simplex and typically does not resolve. A nevus flamus that involves

the ophthalmic and/or maxillary region should alert the examiner to the possibility of Sturge-Weber Syndrome.

- Dermal melanoses are quite common. They were formerly referred to as "Mongolian Spots." They represent increased areas of melanocytes and generally fade as the child ages. It is important not to mistake these for bruises.

References

1. Bland RD. The Newborn Infant. In: Rudolph CD, Rudolph AM, et al. editors. Rudolph's Pediatrics, 21st edition, New York: McGraw-Hill; 2003. p. 55-222.
2. Hay WW, Levin MJ, Sondheimer JM, et al., editors, *Current Diagnosis and Treatment in Pediatrics*, 18th edition, New York: Lange Medical Books/ McGraw-Hill; 2007.
3. Jones KL, *Smith's Recognizable Patterns of Human Malformation.* Philadelphia: Saunders; 1997.
4. Fleisher GR, Ludwig S, Henretig FM, editors. *Textbook of Pediatric Emergency Medicine*, 5th edition, Philadelphia: Lippincott Williams and Wilkins; 2006
5. Gunn, VL, Nechyba C, *The Harriet Lane Handbook*, 17th edition, Philadelphia: Mosby; 2005.

Non-Traumatic Orthopedics

Anne Richter, MD
Department of Emergency Medicine
The University of Arizona

Osteomyelitis

Critical Knowledge

- Bone infection usually caused by hematogenous spread.
- S. *aureus* is the most common organism.
- Treatment requires antibiotics and rarely surgery.

Background

- Fifty percent of cases occur in children age 0-5 years.
- Infection occurs in 3 ways: 1) hematogenous spread is most common in children; 2) contiguous spread of infection after trauma or surgery is less common; 3) infection due to vascular insuffiency is rare in children.
- Any bone may be affected but the femur and tibia are the most common sites.
- S. *aureus* causes the majority of infections with **M**ethicillin – **R**esistant **S**. ***A**ureus* (**MRSA**) increasing nationwide. Other organisms include Strep species, Gram negatives and H. flu. (Table2).

Differential Diagnosis/Critical Concepts

- Suspect osteomyelitis in children with fever, malaise, and bone pain. Swelling and point tenderness are often present.
- Differential Diagnosis (Table 1)
- Work-up
    - Blood culture - positive in 50% of children
    - CBC - white blood cells normal or elevated
    - **E**rythrocyte **S**edimentation **R**ate (**ESR**) and **C** - **R**eactive **P**rotein (**CRP**) - usually increased although may be normal especially in neonates and children with sickle cell disease
    - X-ray often normal for several days after onset of symptoms. Soft tissue swelling may be seen in the first days of illness. Periosteal elevation and bone destruction usually takes 10-21 days to be seen.
    - Bone scan or MRI - bone scan usually shows increased uptake within

48-72 hours of symptoms onset. Advantages of the bone scan include decreased cost, ability to see multiple foci and no sedation is needed. MRI is preferred if pelvic or vertebral infection is suspected, surgical intervention is necessary or abscess is suspected.

Treatment

- Orthopedic consultation
- Surgery rarely needed in cases of osteomyelitis caused by hematogenous spread. Surgery is needed if infection caused by contiguous spread or infection is not improving on antibiotics.
- Antibiotic treatment
  - MRSA not suspected: *nafcillin* or *oxacillin* plus *cefotaxime* or *ceftriaxone*
  - MRSA suspected: *vancomycin* plus *cefotaxime* or *cetriaxone*

Questions

1. What organism is a common cause of osteomyelitis in children with sickle cell disease?
   A. Streptococcus species
   B. Staphlococcus aureus
   C. Staphlococcus epidermidis
   D. Salmonella

   Answer: B. (Although S. aureus is still the most common cause of osteomyelitis in children with sickle cell disease, Salmonella causes a significant number in infections.)

References

1. Lew DP, Waldvogel FA. *Osteomyelitis.* Lancet 2004; 364-79.
2. Gutierrez K. *Bone and Joint Infections in Children.* Pediatr Clin N Amer 2005; 52: 779-94.
3. Blyth MJ, Kincaid R, Craigen MA, Bennet GC. *The changing epidemiology of acute and subacute haematogenous osteomyelitis in children.* J Bone and Joint Surg Br 2001; 83: 99-102.
4. Martinex-Aguilar G, Avalos-MishaanA, HultenK, et al. Community-acquired methicillin-resistant and methicillin susceptible Staphylococcus aureus musculoskeletal infections in children. *Pediatr Infect Dis J* 2004; 23:701-706.

5. Yagupsky P. *Kingella kingae*: from medical rarity to an emerging paediatric pathogen. Lancet Infct Dis 2004;4:358-67.
6. Dagan R. Management of acute haematogenous osteomyelitis and septic arthritis in the pediatric patient. *Pediatr Infect Dis J* 1993;12:88-93.
7. Jaramillo D, Treves S, Kasser J, Harper M, Sundel R, Laor T. Osteomyelitis and Septic Arthritis in Children: Appropriate Use of Imaging to Guide Treatment. *AJR* 1995;165:399-403.

Septic Arthritis

Critical Knowledge

- Serious infection of the joint space most commonly caused by *S. aureus*
- Can be difficult to distinguish from transient synovitis
- Requires rapid diagnosis and treatment with antibiotics and often operative drainage

Background

- Most common in children age 0-3 years
- Can occur in any joint, but most commonly occurs in 1) knee, 2) hip, and 3) elbow
- Bacteria invade the joint most often by hematogenous spread, but can also occur by direct extension, or from inoculation (arthrocentesis or venipucture)
- Organisms causing septic arthritis vary with the age of the patient. (Table 2)
- Before Hib vaccine, *hemophilus influenzae* was a common pathogen

Differential Diagnosis/Critical Concepts

- Difficult to diagnose. Clinical presentation is subtle especially in younger children.
- Clinical manifestations include fever, malaise, guarding of a limb, limp, erythema, swelling, warmth, and pain with passive range of motion.
- Differential diagnosis (Table 1)
- Work-up includes: x-ray, cbc, **E**rythrocyte **S**edimentation **R**ate (**ESR**), blood cultures, ultrasound, arthrocentesis.
- If *N. gonorrhoeae* is suspected cultures of blood, joint fluid, pharynx, cervix and rectum should be obtained.
- Differentiating septic arthritis from transient synovitis (Table 3)

- Radiologic Imaging
  - X-rays may show increase in joint space or bulging of soft tissue
    - Not sensitive for detection of septic arthritis
    - Used to rule out trauma, legg-calves perthes, slipped capital femoral epiphysis, osgood schlatter or malignancy
  - Ultrasound is used to diagnose joint effusion and guide needle aspiration.
  - Arthrocentesis is the most important diagnostic tool
  - Fluid analysis suggestive of septic arthritis
    - Cell count >50,000/mm^3 with >80% neutrophils
    - Gram stain - diagnostic for infection, negative gram stain does not rule out septic arthritis
    - *Glucose* - decreased to 30% of serum
    - Culture - can be negative 1/3 of patients with septic arthritis

Treatment

- Antibiotic treatment
  - Base antibiotic choice on gram stain results if available.
  - If gram stain results are not available, antibiotic choice is the same as osteomyelitis recommendations.
- Surgical therapy
- Obtain prompt orthopedic consult.
- Joint must be adequately drained in order for infection to improve.

Questions

An 8 month-old male infant presents with increased irritability, low-grade fever and will not move his right le.g., No obvious swelling, redness or warmth is present. X-ray is within normal limits. Laboratory values are as follows WBC = 18,000 mm^3, Sed rate= 50mm/hr, Blood culture is pending.

1. What would be your next step in evaluating this patient?
   A. IV antibiotics/call pediatric consultant for admission.
   B. Lumbar puncture
   C. Parenteral antibiotics/next day out-patient follow-up
   D. Ultrasound of hip to evaluate for effusion.
   Answer: D

Questions

1. What diagnostic studies should be ordered to differentiate transient synovitis from a septic joint?
   A. CBC, CRP, x-ray
   B. CBC, Sed Rate, ultrasound and possible arthrocentesis
   C. CBC, BMP, MRI
   D. Sed rate, CRP, bone scan
   Answer: B
2. What treatment is recommended for children with transient synovitis?
   A. Supportive care including pain control with NSAIDS and close follow up with pediatrician
   B. Pain control, antibiotics and close follow up with pediatrician
   C. Casting and outpatient orthopedic referral
   D. Admission with prompt orthopedic referral
   Answer: A

References

1. Bickerstaff DR, Neal LM, Brennan PO, Vell MJ. An investigation into the etiology of irritable hip. *Clin Pediatr* 1991;30:353-6.
2. Hart J. Transient Synovitis of the Hip in Children. *Amer Fam Phys* 1996; 1587-91.
3. Tolat V, Carty H, KlonermanL, Hart CA. *Evidence for a viral aetiology of transient synovitis of the hip.* J Bone and Joint Surg Br 1993;973-4.
4. Haueisen DC, Weiner DS, Weiner SD. The characterization of "transient synovitis of the hip" in children. *J Pedatr Orthop* 1986;6:11-7.
5. Del Beccaro MA, Champoux AN, Bockers T, Mendelman PM. Septic arthritis versus transient synovitis of the hip: the value of screening laboratory tests. *Ann Emerg Med* 1992; 21:1418-22.
6. Kocher MS, Zurakowski D, Kasser JR. Differentiating between septic arthritis and transient synovitis of the hip in children: an evidence-based clinical prediction algorithm. *J bone Joint Surg Am* 1999;81:1662-70.
7. Zawin JK, Hoffer F, Rand F et al. Joint Effusion in Children with an Irritable Hip: US Diagnosis and Aspiration. *Radiology*;187:459-461.

Slipped Capital Femoral Epiphysis

Critical Knowledge

- Displacement of the femoral head on the femoral neck caused by growth disturbance of the proximal femoral growth plate.
- Should be suspected in an obese adolescent child who complains of hip, thigh or knee pain.
- Prompt recognition and orthopedic consult are necessary in order to prevent further slipping which can lead to permanent deformity and arthritis.

Background

- Most common in overweight adolescents during growth spurt (girls age 10-14, boys age 12-15).
- Occurs bilaterally in 25% of children with SCFE.
- Acute slips occur when traumatic force displaces the femoral head and account for 25% of cases.
- Chronic slips occur when no trauma is identified and are thought to be caused by genetics, hormones and increased shear forces.

Differential Diagnosis/Critical Concepts

- Acute slips present with a painful hip held in external rotation and decreased range of motion.
- Chronic slips are harder to diagnose. Can present with vague complaints including hip, groin or knee pain often associated with exercise. External rotation of the hip with flexion is highly suspicious for SCIFE.

Diagnosis

X-ray – need AP view of pelvis and frog-leg of the affected hip. Earliest finding on x-ray is widening of the growth plate. On AP look for Klein's line. Draw a line along the border of femoral neck. On normal hip, line intersects a portion of the femoral head. In SCFE femoral head is below the line. On frog leg view femoral head is medial and posterior to the femoral neck.

Treatment

- Non weight bearing
- Urgent orthopedic referral – pinning in-situ is the treatment of choice.
- If left untreated slipping continues and results in deformity, arthritis and avascular necrosis.

Questions

1. What is the earliest radiograph change associated with SCFE? (Widened blurred growth plate)
   A. Epiphysis posterior to metaphysic
   B. Widened blurred growth plate
   C. Periosteal proliferation of the epiphysis
   D. Premature fusion of the growth plate

   Answer: B (Widened growth plate is the earliest finding followed by answer A. C and D are chronic changes associated with SCFE.)
2. Which view is most sensitive for detecting SCFE?
   A. AP
   B. Lateral
   C. Frog leg AP
   D. Frog leg lateral

   Answer: D (The femoral head displaces medially and posterior to the femoral neck.)

References

1. Perron AD, Miller MD, Brady WJ: Orthopedic Pitfalls in the ED: Slipped Capial Femoral Epiphysis. *J Emerg Med* 2002;20:484-7.
2. Causey AL, Smith ER, Donaldson JJ et al: Missed slipped capital femoral epiphysis: Illustrative cases and review. *J Emerg Med* 1995;13: 175-189.
3. Richards BS: Slipped capital femoral epiphysis. *Pediatr Rev* 1996;17:69-70.
4. Kelsey JL, Acheson RM, Keggi KJ: The body build of patients with slipped capital femoral epiphysis. *Am J Dis Child* 1972;124:276-281.
5. Weiner D: Pathogenesis of slipped capital femoral epiphysis: Current concepts. *J pediatr Orthop* 1996;5:67-73.
6. Rattey T, Piehl F, Wright JG: Acute slipped capital femoral epiphysis; a review of outcomes and rates of avascular necrosis. *J bone Joint Surg Am* 1996;78:398-402.
7. Klein A, Joplin RJ, Reidy JA: Roentgenographic features of slipped apical femoral epiphysis. *Am J Radiol* 1951;66:361-365.
8. Carney BT: *Natural history of untreated chronic slipped capital femoral epiphysis*. Clin Orthop 1996;322:43-47.

Osgood Schlatter Disease

Critical Knowledge

- Benign knee condition consisting of pain and edema of the tibial tubercle occurring in adolescents.
- Treatment includes limiting activities which are pain provoking, and taking NSAIDS.

Background

- A benign condition thought to be caused during periods of rapid growth. Contraction of the quadriceps causes repetitive stress on the patellar tendon, which is transmitted to tibial tubercle causing micro avulsions and inflammation of the tubercle.
- Occurs most often in athletic adolescents (girls age 10-12) and (boys age 12-14) undergoing rapid growth.

Differential Diagnosis/Critical Concepts

- Usually presents as chronic intermittent knee pain. Pain is worse with activity, especially jumping, running and squatting and improved with rest.
- On physical exam soft tissue edema and tenderness of the tibial tubercle are present. Pain is reproduced by extension against resistance. Knee exam is otherwise normal with full range of motion.
- Diagnosis is primarily clinical. Lab tests are not needed unless there is concern for other diagnosis. X-rays are recommended to rule out other etiologies. X-rays may be normal or show prominence or calcification of the tibal tuberosity.

Treatment

- Avoid activities that cause pain- especially jumping and running until pain has been gone for 2-4 months.
- NSAIDS
- Rest, ice compression, elevation
- Once pain has subsided exercises that strengthen hamstrings and increase quadriceps flexibility may help prevent recurrence.
- If symptoms do not improve with conservative treatment, patient should follow up with orthopedics. Surgery is rarely indicated.

Questions

1. True or false: Osgood-Schlatter can be ruled out clinically if a child presents with bilateral intermittent knee pain?

   Answer: False. Approximately 25% of patients with Osgood-Schlatter disease present with bilateral knee pain.

2. How long does a child with Osgood-Schlatter disease need to restrict their activity?

   A. 2-4 weeks

   B. 2-4 weeks after pain is gone

   C. 2-4 months

   D. 2-4 months after pain is gone

   Answer: D

3. Which activities are most likely to cause pain?

   A. Deep knee bends

   B. Descending stairs

   C. Running and jumping

   D. All of the above

   Answer: D

References

1. Bloom OJ, Mackler L, BarbeeJ: Clinical inquiries. What is the best treatment of Osgood-Schlatter disease?. *J of Fam Pract* 2004;53:153 6.
2. Dunn JF: Osgood-Schlatter disease. Am Fam Physician 1990;41:173-6.
3. Krause BL, Williams JP, Catterall A: Natural history of Osgood-Schlatter disease. *J Pediatr Orthop* 1990; 10: 65-8.
4. Smith JB: *Knee problems in children.* Pediatr Clin North Am 1986; 33: 1439-56.
5. Hussain A, Hagroo GA: Osgood-Schlatter disease. *Sports Exer Injury* 1996; 2:202-6.

Legg-Calves Perthes Disease

Critical Knowledge

- Idiopathic osteonecrosis of the femoral head.
- Suspect **L**egg **C**alves **P**erthes **D**isease (**LCPD**) in children 3-12 years old presenting with insidious onset of limp, hip and or knee pain.
- Children with LCPD should be made non-weight bearing and referred to orthopedist.

Background

- Osteonecrosis of the capital femoral epiphysis thought to be caused by vascular occlusion of the femoral head, which makes it more vulnerable to subchondral fracture. Ischemia, infarction and eventual necrosis ensue.
- Occurs most often in boys (5:1 male predominance) age 4-8 years old.
- Seen bilaterally in 10% of children

Differential Diagnosis/Critical Concepts

- Usually presents with painless limp or intermittent hip and knee pain lasting weeks to months.
- Physical exam reveals decreased range of motion with internal rotation and abduction and atrophy of thigh musculature. Positive roll test is elicited when examiner invokes guarding or muscle spasm with internal rotation. Leg length discrepancy is seen in severe disease and suggests total collapse of femoral head.
- Diagnosis includes exclusion of infectious etiologies with CBC, Sed Rate, CRP and occasional arthrocentesis.
- Plain radiographs can establish diagnosis but are often normal early in disease process. Five radiographic stages can be seen on X-ray: 1) cessation of growth- smaller femoral head epiphysis, 2) subchondral fracture- linear lucency in femoral head epiphysis, 3) resorption of bone, 4) re-ossification of new bone, and 5) healed
- More severe course expected if >50% of femoral head involved.
- Bone scan and MRI useful for early diagnosis of LCPD.

Treatment

- Goal of treatment include eliminating hip irritability, restoring normal range of motion, containment of femoral head within acetabulum and maintaining round femoral head.

- Refer child to orthopedist.
- Non-operative treatment includes physical therapy, crutches, and abduction bracing.
- Surgery reserved for severe disease.
- Complications of LCPD include femoral head deformity and degenerative joint disease.

Questions

1. Which of the following are associated with poor prognosis following LCPD?
   A. Age greater than 9 at time of diagnosis
   B. Greater than 50% involvement of the femoral head
   C. Flattened femoral head
   D. All of the above

   Answer: D. Older age, increased involvement of the femoral head and misshapen femoral head (not round) are all associated with poor prognosis for limited range of motion and early development of degenerative joint disease.

2. A six year old boy presents to the emergency department complaining of left hip pain for 3 weeks. Pain is worse with activity and better with rest. Roll sign is positive. A pelvic x-ray is performed which reveals a subchondral fracture. What is the next step in management of this patient?
   A. Make non-weight bearing and refer to orthopedist
   B. Inpatient admission
   C. CBC, Sed rate, CRP, blood culture and ultrasound
   D. MRI

   Answer: A. A subchondral fracture indicates the child has LCPD. No further emergency department work up is necessary. If the x-rays were normal it would be important to rule out infectious etiology for hip pain and should include cbc, sed rate, crp, blood culture and ultrasound. If these tests were negative and symptoms had been occurring for longer than 10 days referral to pcp for bone scan or MRI would be appropriate.

References

1. Roy DR. Current Concepts in Legg-Calve Perthes disease. *Pediatr Ann* 1999 ;28: 748-52.
2. Archives of Disease in Childhood: Epidemiology of Perthes' disease. *Arch Dis Child* 2000;82:385.
3. Salter RB, Thompson GH. Legg-Calve-Perthes disease: the prognostic significance of subchondral fracture and a two-group classification of femoral head involvement. *J Bone Joint Surg Am.* 1984;66:479-489.
4. Kaniklides C. *Diagnostic radiology in Legg-Calve-Perthes disease.* Acta Radiol Suppl 1996;406:1-28.
5. Kaniklides C, Lonnerholm T, Moberg, A. *Legg-Calve-Perthes disease. Comparison of conventional radiography, bone scintigraphy and arthrography.* Acta Radiol 1995;36:434-9.
6. Herring JA. The treatment of Legg-Calve-Perthes disease: a critical review of the literature. *J Bone Joint Surg Am.* 1994;76:448-458.

Other Causes for Limping in Children

Critical Knowledge

There are several other conditions that can present with limping and joint pain in children. These include but are not limited to rheumatic fever (RF), juvenile rheumatoid arthritis (JRA), systemic lupus, erythematous (SLE), Lyme disease and neoplasm. It is important to have a broad differential so as not to miss a critical diagnosis.

Background

- RF is a complication from untreated streptococcal infection that causes damage to connective tissue of heart, joints and blood vessels. Morbidity related to cardiac and neurologic complications. Common in school age children.
- JRA is an autoimmune disease that can cause inflammatory arthritis and is most common in girls age 4-10 years
- SLE involves generation of autoantibodies, which leads to inflammation of microvasculature and multi- organ system involvement. Most common in females of childbearing age.
- Lyme disease is caused by the spirochete, *Borrelia burgdorferi* which is transmitted by Ixodes ticks and found predominantly in the Northeastern

United States. Most commonly seen in children 5-9 years old but can occur at any age.

- Common musculoskeletal tumors in children include rhabdomyosarcoma, osteosarcoma, and Ewing's sarcoma. Rhabdomyosarcoma most common in children less than 10 years old. Osteosarcoma is most common during adolescents while Ewings sarcoma common in children 10-20 years old.

Differential Diagnosis/Critical Knowledge

- Joint involvement in RF occurs early in the disease. Symptoms range from mild arthralgia to migratory arthritis with redness, swelling and extreme pain. Usually associated with fever. Diagnosis based on Jones criteria. No specific confirmatory lab but a positive Streptococcal antibody test helps support the diagnosis. Synovial fluid may have elevated WBC but no organisms.
- JRA presents with acute or insidious joint pain in one or more joints. Intermittent fevers and evanescent rash accompany systemic JRA. Diagnosis depends on clinical findings of arthritis in one or more joints for greater than 6 weeks with other causes excluded. ESR is usually elevated. CBC can reveal lymphopenia and occasional thrombocytopenia. ANA and Rheumatoid factor positive 25% and 20% respectively.
- Acute lymphocytic leukemia often presents with arthritis and can be difficult to distinguish from JRA. The presence of lymphocytosis and neutropenia and thrombocytopenia raises suspicion for leukemia.
- SLE presents most commonly with arthralgia, myalgias and arthritis. Small joints of hands, wrists and knees often involved. Other complaints include fever, malaise, malar rash, renal disease, and many other multi system complaints. Diagnosis based on a series of clinical and laboratory findings. Screening labs should include CBC, BMP, UA, ANA, Anti-dsDNA.
- Suspect Lyme disease in a child who has acute arthritis and has been in an endemic area. Arthritis usually begins as a migratory polyarthritis that develops into monoarticular process involving the knee or ankle. Without treatment episodes last approximately one week and can recur. Chronic arthritis develops in 10 % of patients. Lyme disease can affect multiple organ systems. Diagnosis includes an antibody titer and a confirmatory Western blot test.
- Rhabdomyosarcoma should be suspected in a child with painless soft tissue mass at any site. Osteosarcoma and Ewing's sarcoma most often present with pain or swelling in a bone or joint. Work-up for a suspected bone tumor

should include x-ray, cbc, esr, crp, alkaline phosphatase, electrolytes, joint aspiration. Children need immediate referral to orthopedics and oncologist.

Treatment

- RF prevented by early antibiotic treatment of Strep infections. Once diagnosed NSAIDS to decrease inflammation and appropriate referral to rheumatology, cardiology, or neurology.
- Treatment of JRA includes referral to rheumatologist. Drug regimens can include NSAIDS, *methotrexate*, *etanercept* and *steroids*.
- Treatment of SLE involves specialty referrals, NSAIDS and immunosuppressive drugs. Fever necessitates inpatient admission.
- Antibiotic treatment is recommended for arthritis caused by Lyme disease. Recommended antibiotics include *doxycycline* for children older than 8 years, *amoxicillin* for younger children
- Treatment for pediatric bone tumors includes a combination of chemotherapy, surgical resection and radiation.

Questions

1. A 7 year old female presents with multiple painful joints. She is otherwise health but does report having sore throat and fever 2 weeks previously. What is the most likely diagnosis?

   Answer: Rheumatic fever

2. What other diagnostic criteria is needed to make a diagnosis of rheumatic fever?

   Answer: Jones criteria is used to make the diagnosis of RF. In order to diagnosed RF a patient must have either 1 required evidence plus 2 major criteria and 0 minor criteria or 1 required evidence plus 1 major criteria and 2 minor criteria.

   Required Evidence: evidence of antecedent Strep infection: ASO, Strep antibodies, Strep group A throat culture, recent scarlet fever, anti-deoxyribonuclease B, anti-hyaluronidase

   Major Criteria: carditis, polyarthritis, chorea, erythema marginatum, subcutaneous nodules

   Minor Criteria: fever, arthralgia, previous rheumatic fever, acute phase reactants (CRP, Sed Rate, leukocytosis), prolonged pr interval

Table 1: Differential Diagnosis for a Limping Child by Age	
All Ages Septic Arthritis Osteomyelitis Cellulitis Neoplasm	**Age 4-10** Legg-Calves Perthes Transient synovitis Arthritis (JRA, Lyme disease, RF) Fracture
Age 1-3 Arthritis (JRA, Lyme disease) Osgood Schlatter Arthritis (Lyme disease, SLE, gonococcal)	**Age 11-16** Slipped capital femoral Developmental dysplasia of the hip Leg-length discrepancy Foreign body in the foot

Table 2: Most Common Organisms Causing Septic Arthritis		
Age 0-2 Months	**Age 2 months to 5 years**	**Age >5 years**
Staph aureus	Staph aureus	Staph aureus
Group B Strep	Strep pyogenes	Strep pyogenes
Gram negative enterococci	Strep. pneumoniae	Neisseria gonorrhoeae
N. gonorrhoeae	Kingella kingae	

Table 3: Differentiating Septic Arthritis from Transient Synovitis: 4 Predictors	
Predictors of Septic Arthritis	**Predicted Probability of Septic Arthrits**
History of Fever	0-predictors = 0.1% probability septic arthritis
Non-weight Bearing	1-predictor= 2.1-5.3% probability septic arthritis
Sed Rate >40mm/h	2-predictors= 33.8-62.2% probability septic arthritis
Serum WBc >12,000/mm^3	3-predictors= 93-95.2% percent probability septic arthritis
	4-predictors= 99.8% probability septic arthritis

References

1. Adams, Lehman TJ. Update on the pathogenesis and treatment of systemic onset juvenile rheumatoid arthritis. Curr Opin Rheumatol 2005;17:612-6. Ilowite NT. Current treatment of juvenile rheumatoid arthritis. *Pediatrics* 2002; 109: 109-15.
2. Birdi N, Hosking M, Clulow MK, et al. Acute rheumatic fever and post streptococcal reactive arthritis: diagnostic and treatment practices of pediatric subspecialists in Canada. *J Rheumatol* 2001;28: 1681-8.
3. Warren RW, Perez MD, Wilking AP, Myones BL. *Pediatric rheumatic diseases.* Pediatr Clin North Am 1994; 41: 783-818. Edworthy SM. Clinical Manifestations of Systemic Lupus Erythematosus. In: Harris ED, et al, Eds. Kelley's Textbook of Rheumatology, 7th Editions. Saundres, 2005; 1201-1224.
4. Bartels CM, Hildebrand J, Mueller D. Systemic Lupus Erythematosus. *Emedicine* 2006.
5. Nadelman RB, Wormser GP. Lyme Borreliosis. Lancet 1998; 352: 557-65. Steere AC. Lyme disease. *N Engl J Med* 1989; 321: 586-96.
6. Carola AS, Arndt MD and Crist WM. Common Musculoskeletal Tumors of Childhood and Adolescence. *N Engl J of Med* 1999; 341:342-351.
7. Kocher et al. Differentiating Between Septic Arthritis and Transient Synovitis of the Hip in Children: An Evidence Based Clinical Prediction Algorithm. *The Journal of Bone and Joint Surgery* 1999 81: 1662-70.

Orthopedic Trauma

Drew Watters, MD
Department of Emergency Medicine
The University of Arizona

Critical Knowledge

- Understand the differences that age imparts on anatomy, physiology, and pathology
- Preverbal children cannot describe the bones that are injured
- In general, children will not use an injured limb. Look for a limb that the child does not move, or "self-splints" by holding
- Look for overlying signs associated with fractures. Fully move all joints to ensure there are no dislocations or areas of tenderness. Be sure to assess femurs and pelvis, as these fractures may be rapidly life threatening
- Treat pain appropriately. It is appropriate to use narcotics to treat pain in children

Background and Anatomy

- Pediatric orthopedic injuries are commonly seen in urgent cares, emergency departments, and outpatient clinics
- Children have relatively more pliability, which means a lot more damage can be done to soft tissue without associated fracture
- Children have growth plates and ossification centers that fuse as they age, and their smaller muscle mass can increase risks for ligament injuries and dislocations
- Pliable bones lead to different fractures than adults

Differential Diagnosis

- Contusion
- Sprain
- Hematoma
- Ligamentous injury
- Dislocation
- Fracture
- Non-traumatic injury/metabolic disease (see "Nontraumatic Orthopedics")

Critical Concepts

Open vs. Closed Fractures

One must immediately determine if a fracture is open, in order to quickly treat it with irrigation, antibiotics, and orthopedic consultation.

Referred Pain

Pain may be felt away from the site of injury, especially in children with limited verbal skills. Complaint of knee pain may stem from hip injury, and vice versa. Shoulder pain can be due to underlying spleen or liver injuries.

Injury type

- Can often be narrowed down based on the mechanism. For example, a fall onto an outstretched hand ("FOOSH") can cause scaphoid, radius, supracondylar fractures, or elbow dislocations.
- Falls with a twisting motion may cause spiral fractures. A fall onto a bent elbow can cause an olecranon fracture.
- Being tackled from the side can cause the "unhappy triad" of ACL, medial meniscus, and MCL tears.
- Fractures in athletes, especially runners, are often due to chronic, repetitive stress.

Treatment

- Will vary by injury, but should always include pain control
- Disposition planning should include consideration
  - The child's safety
  - The need for a wheelchair, crutches, assistance, and limitations
  - A follow-up plan to see an orthopedist or PCP, if necessary
  - Instructions to return with worsening signs or symptoms
  - Instructions on fracture care at home
- Serious injuries or multiple injuries may warrant admission for observation

Questions

1. Which of the following fractures is potentially fatal?
   A. Tibia
   B. Femur
   C. Humerus

D. Ulna

Answer: B, Femur fractures and pelvic fractures may lead to shock and death. Immediate diagnosis and treatment of these injuries is essential. All the other fractures are not fatal but may be associated with or lead to severe limb damage.

Nursemaid's Elbow

Critical Concepts

- A subluxation of the radial head under the annular ligament
- Often mistaken for a true fracture
- Classically caused by pulling or lifting a toddler by an outstretched hand
- Usually presents with a child unwilling to use the affected arm

Diagnosis

- Anxiety is often greater than pain
- Arm is often held in 15-20 degrees of flexion, often supported by the other arm.
- Bruising, redness, or signs of trauma are absent

Treatment

- Easily treated without radiographs, if there is no concern for coexisting injury
- Reduced by hyper-pronation of the hand, extension, and then flexion at the elbow
- If unable to reduce the dislocation after 2-3 attempts, X-rays should be obtained
- Families should be counseled that recurrence is common, and educated to avoid axial traction

Dislocations

Critical Concepts

- Separation of a bone from the joint in which it normally rests
- May be associated with fractures or neurovascular injuries
- May include ligament or tendon damage
- Require manipulation and reduction to restore function
- If unreduced, may cause permanent injury to joint, nerves, and bones

- Always assess nerve and vascular function before and after reduction

Diagnosis

- Differential includes ligamentous injury, muscle injury, or fracture
- Abnormal contours of the joint may be seen or felt
- Extremity may rotated, of irregular length, or non-functional
- Range of motion will by limited due to joint disruption
- Radiographs are warranted to evaluate for associated fractures
- Assess nerve and vascular function to ensure no compromise

Treatment

- After initial assessment, pain should be managed, and muscle relaxers may aid reduction. Successful reduction may require sedation.
- Specific reduction varies by affected joint, and there are myriad techniques
- Reduction often requires a large force, but avoid sudden motions that may cause injury
- In general, the joint should be realigned with gentle traction, rotating the joint the free the dislocated bone from entrapment
- After reduction, the joint should be splinted or placed in a sling
- Obtain post-reduction X-rays to ensure reduction and re-assess for fractures
- Reassess the extremity for neurovascular function after splinting

Questions

1. A 16 year old girl presents after diving into a pool from a 3-meter board and complaining of immediate right shoulder pain. She has pain to palpation at the superior, anterior aspect of the shoulder. She cannot abduct the shoulder or range it actively, but it can be (painfully) ranged passively. The best test and most likely diagnosis

   A. X-ray and dislocation

   B. X-ray and AC separation

   C. X-Ray and fracture

   D. CT and dislocation

   E. CT and fracture

   Answer: B, X-ray and separation. The mechanism is most concerning for acromioclavicular (AC) separation versus shoulder dislocation. Her physical exam favors separation, however, because there is no appreciable deformity, she is able to be ranged fully, and she is tender at the AC ligament (which is at the anterior, superior aspect of the shoulder, where the clavicle ends). X-rays should be obtained to rule out dislocation or fractures.

Fractures

Critical Concepts

- Generally the result of trauma, and are often associated with other injuries
- If one fracture is found, assess for others
- Combination fractures of note include
  - Lumbar fractures associated with calcaneous fractures
  - Maisonneuve fracture (medial malleolus fracture with a proximal tibial fracture)
  - Lisfranc fractures (fracture and dislocation of the midfoot)
- If history is unusual for injury, raises concern for underlying pathology or abuse
  - Consider bone cysts, cancer, or osteogenesis imperfecta
  - Assess safety of child and report if there is concern for abuse
- Fractures may be of varying severity, with little or no radiographic evidence

Diagnosis

- Physical exam to localize areas of injury and look for coexistent injuries

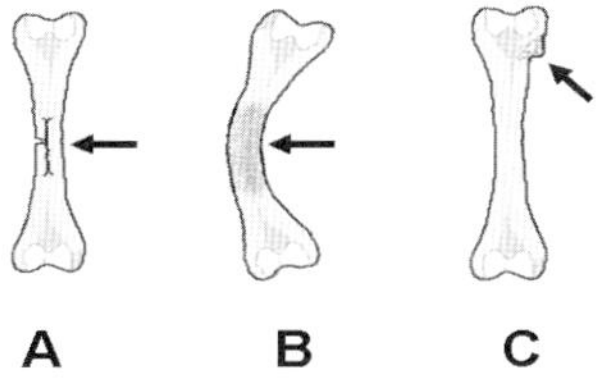

Figure 1: Pediatric Fracture Patterns

A. Greenstick Fracture, arrow demonstrates the direction of force causing the fracture. (Note the fracture line opposite to the side of force along with a vertical fracture component.)

B: Plastic deformity, arrow demonstrates the direction of force causing the fracture.

C: Torus fracture. Arrow demonstrates the buckle deformity in the bony cortex.

- Generally X-rays are needed for complete diagnosis.

- X-ray may show obvious deformity, cortical irregularities, or irregularity in comparison of growth plates
- Subtle findings may include a prominent fat pad. Articular injury can cause lucency between the cortex and surrounding soft tissue; therefore, any obvious lucency along the cortex should be concerning for occult fracture
- Pediatric fractures may have unique patterns (see figure)
  - Torus: buckling of the cortex
  - Greenstick: bending of the bone with unilateral cortex irregularity
  - Plastic deformities: bending of the bone with no cortical irregularities

Treatment

- Femur and pelvic fractures must be diagnosed and treated emergently, as they can cause significant blood loss and shock
- Patient pain should be treated appropriately
- Fractures should be elevated, splinted and cooled as quickly as possible for stability and pain control
- Reduction and splinting should be done as indicate, once definitive diagnosis is made

Questions

1. A 5 year old boy presents after a fall with left thigh pain and bruising laterally. X-rays show curvature of the femur with no irregularity of the cortex. The patient ambulates with complaint of pain in the lateral thigh. Which of the following is the best next step?

   A. Consult orthopedics

   B. Place in a posterior leg splint

   C. If patient is ambulatory, arrange follow-up with orthopedics in 3-5 days

   D. CT the femur

   E. X-ray the contralateral thigh

   Answer: E, X-ray the contralateral thigh. Curvature may represent a plastic deformity, but may also be a normal variation, a result of malnutrition (Rickett's), or evidence of bone malformation. Imaging the contralateral femur will reveal any asymmetry, which would support the diagnosis of fracture.

Pelvic Fracture

Critical Concepts

- Often the result of large forces, and can be fatal
- Often associated with other orthopedic and intra-abdominal injuries
- May be unstable and require immediate treatment

Diagnosis

- Portable X-rays should be obtained immediately if there is concern for fracture
- Be sure to fully palpate and stress the pelvis
- Place your hands on the lateral pelvic wall and compress; press also on the pubic symphysis
- Any instability or deformity requires emergent evaluation and care
- If fracture is found, CT of the abdomen/pelvis is indicated to rule out additional bleeding or injuries
- If the patient is unstable, emergent evaluation by surgery and interventional radiology (if available) is indicated

Treatment

- IV access, pain control, and fluid resuscitation should be initiated
- If instability is felt during primary exam, a pelvic binder should be placed
- If a binder is unavailable, a sheet may be folded, placed around the pelvis, and then tied tightly across the anterior pelvis to hold the fracture
- After binder placement, reassess the pelvis and lower extremities
- Emergent consultation by orthopedic surgery should be made
- If patient is unstable or there is active bleeding, interventional radiology may need to perform embolization

Questions

1. A 15 year old girl is in an MVC and presents intubated and sedated. Primary survey reveals multiple abrasions, contusions, and lacerations. Her pelvis feels stable to examination. She is hypotensive and tachycardic. Which of the following is the most appropriate first step?

   A. X-ray pelvis

   B. Ultrasound abdomen and pelvis

   C. Initiate IV fluids

D. CT abdomen and pelvis

Answer: C, initiate IV fluids. Initial treatment of a trauma patient should not be contingent on diagnostics. Since the patient's airway has been established (patient is intubated) and no active bleeding is found to control, the next step is to manage the hypotension by fluid resuscitation. Initial diagnostics should include X-rays of the chest and pelvis, as well as FAST ultrasound of the abdomen, heart, and pelvis.

Compartment Syndrome

Critical Concepts

- Neurovascular compromise of tissue due to increasing pressure in a contained space, such as the fascia of an extremity
- Be aware of increasing pain, as it is the first symptom
- Failure to treat may lead to limb ischemia, nerve damage, and necrosis

Diagnosis

- Early signs include pain with passive movement of the associated extremity (e.g., forearm pain elicited by passive finger flexion)
- Late signs include pallor, pulselessness, coldness, and paresthesias… Do Not Wait for these signs!
- May be diagnosed by measuring pressures directly in the compartment
- If there is concern, emergent orthopedic consultation should be made

Treatment

- Elevate and ice the area to reduce swelling and prevent increasing pressure
- If compartment syndrome is diagnosed, fasciotomy must be performed
- Incise through the skin and fascia of the affected compartment

Questions

1. A 13 year old boy fell onto his left elbow and suffered a supracondylar fracture. He has diffuse swelling to the arm and severe pain on palpation. Which of the following is the most appropriate initial treatment?

   A. Measure compartment pressures

   B. Administer *Ativan* for pain

   C. Elevate and ice the arm

   D. Consult orthopedics

Answer: C, elevate and ice. This injury is concerning for potential development of compartment syndrome. Elevation, ice, and mild compression help limit swelling and pressure. *Ativan* (*benzodiazepines*) do not treat pain. Orthopedic consultation and pressure monitoring may be indicated, but should be done after initial treatment.

Growth Plate Injuries

Critical Concepts

- Fractures are classified as **S**alter-**H**arris (**SH**) Types I-V (see figure)
    - I- no visible fracture
    - II- fracture through metaphysic only
    - III- fracture through epiphysis only;
    - IV- fracture through both meta- and epiphysis
    - V- crush injury in plate
- Growth plate injuries may lead to nonunion healing, unequal extremities, chronic pain, and myositis ossificans (bone formation in surrounding muscle).
- SH Type V is difficult to diagnose, and may have serious sequelae. You must have a high level of suspicion
- The age of the child affects potential outcome: younger children have higher risk of growth abnormalities

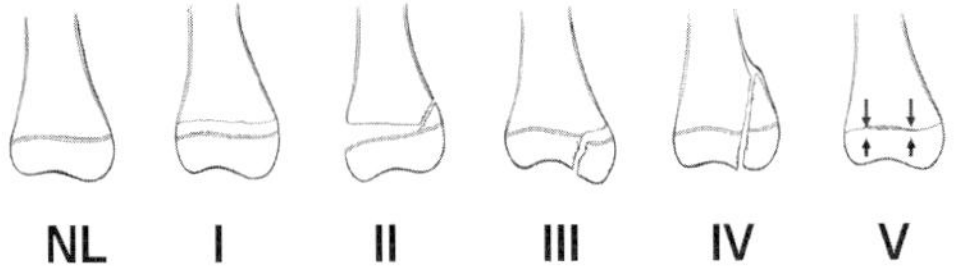

Figure 2: Salter-Harris (SH) Fracture Types

NL: normal physis,
I: type I SH fracture: fracture through the physis
II: type II SH fracture: fracture through the physis and metaphysis
III: type III SH fracture: fracture through the physis and epiphysis
IV: type IV SH fracture: fracture through the physis, metaphysis and epiphsis.
V: type V SH fracture: Crush injury of the physis (arrows demonstrate crush force).

Diagnosis

- Obtain radiographs and assess for evidence and severity of injury
- Compare the growth plate to the contralateral side

- Occasionally CT is required to delineate the extent of injury

Treatment

- Use ice, elevation, and mild compression. Treat pain accordingly
- SH Type I and II fractures may often be treated by splinting and orthopedic follow up in 7-10 days
- SH Types III-V require orthopedic consultation, as they often require surgical fixation

Questions

1. A 7 year old girl fell 12 feet onto her feet, and now complains of severe pain in the right knee. X-rays of the knee are negative. Which of the following is the most appropriate next step?
   A. Place in a posterior splint and follow up with PCP in 7-10 days
   B. Place in knee immobilizer and follow up with PCP in 7-10 days
   C. CT of the knee
   D. MRI of the knee
   E. Discharge patient for follow up with Orthopedist in 7-10 days

   Answer: C, CT of the knee. This patient has a mechanism concerning for crush injury to the growth plate (Salter-Harris Type V). If X-rays are negative but concern is high, further imaging is indicated. MRI, while diagnostic, is more expensive, more difficult to perform, and may not be necessary; it may be ordered in conjunction with orthopedic consultation.

Spinal Injuries

Critical Concepts

- May be life-threatening, causing respiratory failure, paralysis, or shock
- **S**pinal **C**ord **I**njury **W**ithout **R**adiographic **A**bnormality (**SCIWORA**) is not rare
- Clinical suspicion must be high, especially with neurologic signs or symptoms
- Younger children have greater pliability and higher risk of SCIWORA

Diagnosis

- A thorough physical exam is needed to evaluate neurologic function
- X-rays of the pediatric spine may be useful but may miss significant injuries
- CT or MRI is warranted if clinical concern is high or if X-rays are inadequate

Treatment

- Initial treatment by EMS or emergency staff should include spinal immobilization
- Assess and manage the ABCs, with attention to the airway
- Pain and agitation should be treated appropriately
- Evidence of injury warrants emergent evaluation by a spinal surgeon
- Steroid protocol may be initiated, in consultation with a spine surgeon

Questions

1. A 10 year old boy presents in a C-spine collar after a fall. He has rapid, shallow breaths and paralysis of all extremities. Heart rate is 180, blood pressure is 87/43, and respiratory rate is 45. Immediate management of this patient requires which of the following?
   A. Consultation by a spinal surgeon
   B. Initiation of high-dose *steroids*
   C. Morphine for pain
   D. Supplemental oxygen and preparation for intubation
   E. Transfusion of blood

   Answer: D, Cervical spine injuries may lead to paralysis of respiratory muscles and subsequent respiratory failure. Early management of the airway is essential, and may require intubation. Consultation, imaging, and medication initiation should be done after the primary assessment is finished.

References

1. Carson, S, Woolridge, D: *Pediatric Upper Extremity Injuries*. The Pediatric clinics of North America 2006, vol. 53, nº 1
2. Peterson HA: *Physeal & apophyseal injuries*. In: Rockwood CA, Wilkins KE.
3. Beaty JH, eds. *Fractures in Children*. 4th ed. Lippincott-Raven; 1996.
4. Bright RW: *Physeal injuries. In: Fractures: Fractures in Children*. 3rd ed. Lippincott-Raven; 1991: 87-186.
5. Wolfram, W: *Pediatrics, Nursemaid Elbow* Jan 4, 2007. www.emedicine.com
6. Blasier RD, Aronson J, Tursky, EA: External fixation of pediatric femur fractures. *J Pediatr Orthop* 1997 May-Jun; 17(3): 342-6
7. Harrington KD: Orthopaedic management of extremity and pelvic lesions. *Clin Orthop* 1995 Mar; (312): 136-47

8. Kanel JS: Treatment of fractures of the femur in children and adolescents. *West J Med* 1995; 163(6): 570
9. Biffl WL, Smith WR, Moore EE, et al: Evolution of a multidisciplinary clinical pathway for the management of unstable patients with pelvic fractures. *Ann Surg* 2001 Jun; 233(6): 843-50
10. Hart RG, Rittenberry TJ, *Uehara DT: Handbook of Orthopaedic Emergencies.* Lippincott-Raven; 1999: 277-297
11. Blick SS, Brumback RJ, Poka A, et al: Compartment syndrome in open tibial fractures. *J Bone Joint Surg Am* 1986 Dec; 68(9): 1348-53
12. Geller E: *Emergency treatment of the trauma patient.* In: Dee R, Hurst LC, 13. Gruber MA, Kottmeier SA, eds. Principles of Orthopedic Practice. NY: McGraw-Hill; 1997:379-388.
13. McQueen MM, Christie J, Court-Brown CM: Acute compartment syndrome in tibial diaphyseal fractures. *J Bone Joint Surg Br* 1996 Jan; 78(1): 95-8
14. Dabney KW, Lipton G: Evaluation of limp in children. *Curr Opin Pediatr* 1995 Feb; 7(1): 88-94
15. Lee RW, *Demos TC: Limp and altered gait.* In: Rosen P, Doris PE, Berkin RM, et al, eds. Diagnostic Radiology in Emergency Medicine. 1992:509-40
16. Berkowitz CD: Pediatric abuse. New patterns of injury. *Emerg Med Clin North Am* 1995 May; 13(2): 321-41
17. Ludwig S, Kornberg AE, eds: *Child Abuse: A Medical Reference.* 2nd ed. New York: Churchill Livingston; 1992.
18. Sugar NF, Taylor JA, Feldman KW: *Bruises in infants and toddlers: those who don't cruise rarely bruise.* Puget Sound Pediatric Research Network. Arch Pediatr Adolesc Med 1999 Apr; 153(4): 399-403
19. Brown CV, Antevil JL, Sise MJ: Spiral computed tomography for the diagnosis of cervical, thoracic, and lumbar spine fractures: its time has come. *J Trauma* 2005 May; 58(5): 890-5
20. Hadley MN, Walters BC, Grabb PA: Guidelines for the management of acute cervical spine and spinal cord injuries. *Clin Neurosurg* 2002; 49: 407-98[Medline]. 22. Harris MB, Sethi RK: The initial assessment and management of the multiple-trauma patient with an associated spine injury. Spine 2006 May 15; 31(11 Suppl): S9-15
21. Stiell IG, Clement CM, McKnight RD: The Canadian C-spine rule versus the NEXUS low-risk criteria in patients with trauma. *N Engl J Med* 2003 Dec 25; 349(26): 2510-8

Pneumonia

Charles Gillespie, MD
Department of Emergency Medicine/Pediatrics Combined Resident
Department of Emergency Medicine and Pediatrics
The University of Arizona

Critical Actions

- ABCs, IV, O_2, monitor, pulse oximetry, CXR, CBC
- Consider septic workup in very young and/or toxic-appearing patients
- Shortness of breath is NOT always pulmonary in origin: consider cardiac dysrhythmia/dysfunction and congestive heart failure
- Administer empiric antibiotics based on most likely etiologic agents

Background/Epidemiology/Anatomy

- Pneumonia is inflammation of lung tissue from infectious/noninfectious causes
- Risk factors increase incidence
  - Very young (esp. prematurity)
  - Chronically ill or immunosuppressed
  - Malnutrition
  - Tobacco exposure
  - Daycare
- Causative organisms vary with age (Table 1)
  - Viral (60-90%)
    - RSV and parainfluenza are most common
    - Others: influenza, adenovirus, enterovirus, rhinovirus, measles, varicella, rubella, herpes simplex virus, cytomegalovirus, Epstein-Barr virus, hantavirus
  - Bacterial
    - More common in hospitalized children
    - Typicals: Strep. pneumoniae, Staph. aureus, Haemophilus influenzae, Pseudomonas aeruginosa
    - Atypicals: Mycoplasma, Chlamydia pneumoniae
  - Fungal, protozoal, and tuberculosis
    - Consider in chronic pneumonia

        - TB risk factors: urban, immigrant, exposure, immuno-suppressed
- Symptoms in neonates & young infants
    - Lethargy, poor feeding
    - Fever or hypothermia
    - Apnea, flaring, grunting, tachypnea
    - Vomiting, diarrhea
    - Bradycardia and shock
- Symptoms in older children
    - Malaise, headache
    - Fever, chills
    - Cough with sputum production
    - Dyspnea, pleuritic chest pain
- Physical exam signs
    - Fever
    - Tachypnea
    - Tachycardia
    - Tactile fremitus
    - Dullness to percussion
    - Egophony
    - Rales

Diagnostic Evaluation

- CXR
    - Typical findings in a bacterial PNA: consolidation or lobar/segmental infiltrate
    - Typical findings in a viral or atypical bacterial PNA: diffuse, patchy infiltrate, hyperinflation, peribronchial thickening/cuffing
    - Findings may vary and overlap so are not 100% reliable
- CBC
    - Bacterial: ↑WBC count with a left shift (neutrophils)
    - Viral: ↑WBC count with a right shift (lymphocytes)
- Blood culture: positive in ≤10% cases
- C-Reactive Protein: closer correlation with bacteremia & lobar infiltrates than an elevevated WBC count

- Sputum culture
    - May help guide antibiotic therapy, though 50% non-diagnostic
    - Difficult to obtain in small children
- Nasopharyngeal/oropharyngeal culture and gram stain
    - May detect chlamydia, pertussis, mycoplasma
    - Rapid antigen tests for RSV, influenza available
- Consider PPD skin test for suspicion of tuberculosis
- Urine and CSF cultures for neonates at risk for sepsis/meningitis

Differential Diagnosis

- Allergic alveolitis
- Aspiration pneumonitis
- Atelectasis
- Bronchopulmonary dysplasia
- Chronic pulmonary disease (cystic fibrosis, asthma)
- Coccidiomycosis
- Congenital heart disease/CHF
- Congenital pulmonary abnormalities
- Empyema
- Foreign body aspiration
- Pneumatocele
- Pneumothorax
- Misinterpreted radiological study
- Neoplasm
- Tuberculosis

Critical Concepts

- With treatment, most uncomplicated bacterial pneumonia improves in 1-2 days
- Immunizations dramatically decrease the incidence of Haemophilus Influenaze Type B & and Strep. pneumoniae
- Bacterial pneumonia may be preceded by viral upper respiratory infections
- RSV pneumonia rarely occurs with bacterial co-infection

- For recurrent pneumonia, investigate underlying causes
  - Abnormal secretions/clearance (CF, asthma, ciliary dyskinesia)
  - Airway obstruction (foreign body, vascular ring, malignancy)
  - Aspiration susceptibility (gastroesophageal reflux, vocal cord paralysis, etc.)
  - Congenital heart disease (especially those with L→R shunt lesions)
  - Immunodeficiency
  - Pulmonary anomalies (bronchopulmonary dysplasia, pulmonary sequestration, tracheoesophageal fistula, tracheal stenosis)
- Remember that infiltrates on CXR may persist for weeks to months following resolution of illness

Treatment

- Treat hypoxia with supplemental oxygen
- Treat dehydration with IVF (tachypnea increases insensible water loss)
- Treat fever with *acetaminophen/ibuprophen*
- Consider bronchodilators for significant bronchospasm/wheezing
- Treat empirically with antibiotics based on age and suspected etiology (Table 2)

Disposition

- Most cases treated on outpatient basis with close follow up in 1-2 days
- Admission considerations
  - Children <3mos
  - History of apnea, cyanosis, desaturation with crying, feeding or exertion
  - Underlying lung disease or prematurity
  - Children who appear toxic, dyspneic or hypoxic (<90-93% SaO2 @ S.L.)
  - Children who cannot tolerate PO fluids or medications
  - Evidence of significant pleural effusion on CXR
  - Suspected bacterial pneumonia in infants (especially multilobar involvement)
  - Suspected aspiration pneumonia (higher likelihood of progression)
  - Suspected staphlococcal or Hib pneumonia (e.g., pneumatocele on CXR)

- Poor response to outpatient therapy within 24-48 hrs
- Unsupportive family situation

Table 1: Common Etiologies of Pediatric Pneumonia

Age	Organism	Comments
Neonates (<28 days)	Bacteria Group B streptococcus *Listeria, E. coli* Viruses	Neonates: bacterial >viral causes due to aspiration of maternal flora during birth
2 wks – 2 mos	Viruses Bacteria *Strep. pneumo* *Staph. aureus* *Chlamydia* *Haemophilus* (HIB & nontype B)	*Chlamydia*: afebrile pneumonitis with staccato cough & rales in otherwise well infant
2 mos – 3 yrs	Viruses Bacteria *Strep. pneumo* *Staph. aureus* *Haemophilus* (HIB & nontype B)	*Hib* infections ⇓ 99% after conjugate vaccines introduced; asymptomatic colonization with nontype B is common (40-80%)
3 yrs – 12 yrs	Viruses Bacteria *Strep. pneumo* *Mycoplasma*	*S. pneumo* infections ⇓ 80% after PCV7 vaccines introduced; high risk pts include sickle-cell, HIV, asplenia, cochlear implant
13 yrs – 19 yrs	Viruses Bacteria *Strep. Pneumo* *Mycoplasma*	*Mycoplasma pneumomiae* most common etiology in school aged children, esp 10-15 yrs

Table 2: Common Therapies for Pediatric Pneumonia		
Patient Characteristics	**Inpatient Therapy (IV)**	**Outpatient Therapy (PO)**
Neonates (<28 days)	*Ampicillin* 50 mg/kg/dose plus *Cefotaxime* 50 mg/kg/dose or *Gentamycin* 2.5 mg/kg/dose	Not Recommended Consider *Acyclovir* 10 mg/kg/dose
1-3 mos (sx of *Chlamydia*)	*Erythromycin** 10 mg/kg/dose *or* *Azithromycin* 2.5 mg/kg/dose if febrile add: *Cefotaxime* 50 mg/kg/dose	*Azithromycin* 10 mg/kg on day one then 5 mg/kg/day x 4 days or *Erythromycin* 10 mg/kg/dose (*reports of hypertrophic pyloric stenosis & V-tach in neonates)
1 mo-5 yrs	*Cefuroxime* 50 mg/kg/dose or *Ampicillin* 50 mg/kg/dose or *Ceftriaxone* 50 mg/kg/dose IM (if poor POs during first 24hrs)	*Amoxicillin* 45 mg/kg/dose or *Azithromycin* 10 mg/kg on day one then 5 mg/kg/day x 4 days
6-18 yrs	*Ceftriaxone* 50 mg/kg/dose or *Cefotaxime* 50 mg/kg/dose plus *Azithromycin* 10 mg/kg/dose	*Azithromycin* 10 mg/kg on day one (500 mg max) then 5 mg/kg x 4 days (250 mg/day max)
Critically ill or suspected resistant *S. pneumoniae*	To std therapy add *Vancomycin* 20 mg/kg/dose	Not Recommended

Patient Characteristics	Inpatient Therapy (IV)	Outpatient Therapy (PO)
Vent-dependent or multiple hospitalizations Suspect *Pseudomonas,* though frequently polymicrobial (e.g., *S. aureus, Klebsiella, E. coli*)	*Ceftazidime* 50 mg/kg/dose or *Cefepime* 50 mg/kg/dose or *Meropenem* 20 mg/kg/dose (MSSA & gram negs) +/- *Vancomycin* 10-15 mg/kg/dose (MRSA)	Not Recommended
Viral pneumonia • Antibiotics not useful • Most resolve with supportive care • May predispose to bacterial infection	HIV Pts with PCP pneumonia TMP-SMX 20 mg/kg/day RSV prophylaxis for infants <24 mos with chronic lung dz or <32wk gestation *Palivizumab* 15 mg/kg/dose IM	Influenza A or B *Oseltamivir* (≥1yo) or *Zanamivir* (≥5yo) May ⇓ duration of illness by 1 day, but not shown to prevent influenza-related complications (i.e., viral or bacterial PNA)

Questions

1. Which organism often produces pneumonia without the symptom of fever?
   - A. Streptococcus pneumoniae
   - B. Bordatella pertussis
   - C. Chlamydia trachomatis
   - D. Mycoplasma pneumoniae

   Answer: C

2. In which age-group do bacterial organisms produce the most cases of pneumonia?
   - A. 0 to 3 wks
   - B. 3 mos to 3 yrs
   - C. 3 to 13 yrs

   Answer: A

3. Case fatality from *pneumococcal* infection are highest in children
   A. With underlying liver disease
   B. With asplenia
   C. With underlying cardiac disease
   D. With cystic fibrosis

   Answers: B

References

1. American Academy of Pediatrics, Committee on Infectious Diseases. Policy Statement: Recommendations for the prevention of *pneumococcal* infections, including the use of *pneumococcal* vaccine (Prevnar), pneuococcal polysaccharide vaccine, and antibiotic prophylaxis. *Pediatrics.* Aug 2000;106:362-366.
2. American Academy of Pediatrics, Committee on Infectious Diseases and Committee on Fetus and Newborn. Policy Statement: Revised Indications for the Use of Palivizumab and Respiratory Syncytial Virus Immune Globulin Intravenous for the Prevention of Respiratory Syncytial Virus Infections. *Pediatrics.* Vol. 112 No. 6 December 2003; pp. 1442-1446.
3. American Academy of Pediatrics, Redbook: Report of the Committee on Infectious Diseases 2006. Section 3: Summaries of Infectious Diseases; pp 310-318, 525-536.
4. Brown, K., Gilford, W.; *Viral and Bacterial Pneumonia in Children.* Emergency Medicine: A Comprehensive Study Guide 6th Ed. Ch 123; pp 784-789.
5. Campbell, S., Marri.e., T., Anstey, R., Dickinson, G., Ackroyd-Stolarz, S.; The Contribution of Blood Cultures to the Clinical Management of Adult Patients Admitted to the Hospital With Community-Acquired Pneumonia. *Chest.* 2003; 123: 1142-1150.
6. Elward, A., Warren, D., Fraser, V.; Ventilator-Associated Pneumonia in Pediatric Intensive Care Unit Patients: Risk Factors and Outcomes. *Pediatrics.* May 2002; 109: 758-764.
7. Fleisher, G.; *Infectious Disease Emergencies: Lower Respiratory Infections.* Textbook of Pediatric Emergency Medicine 5th Ed. Ch 84;pp 809-14.
8. Gaston, B.; *Pediatrics in Review*: Pneumonia. 2002; 23:132-140.
9. Gilbert, D, Moellering, R, Eliopoulos, G, Sande, M., *The Sanford Guide to Antimicrobial Therapy* 2006. Pneumonia in Neonates/Infants/Children; Table 1; pp 28-29.

10. Kimani, K.; *Microbiology and Infectious Disease.* The Harriet Lane Handbook 17th Ed. Ch 16; p 421.
11. Kollef, M., Morrow, L., Niederman, M., Leeper, K., Anzueto, A., Benz-Scott, I., Rodino, F.; Clinical Characteristics and Treatment Patterns Among Patients with Ventilator-Associated Pneumonia Patterns. *Chest.* 2006;129;1210-1218.
12. Michelow, I., Olsen, K., Lozano, J., Rollins, N., Duffy, L., Ziegler, T., Kauppila, J., Leinonen, M., McCracken, G. Epidemiology and Clinical Characteristics of Community-Aquired Pneumonia in Hospitalized Children. *Pediatrics* Vol. 113 No. 4 April 2004; pp. 701-707.
13. Tsutomu Yamazaki, Kei Murayama, Atsuko Ito, Suzuko Uehara, and Nozomu Sasaki. Epidemiology of Community-Acquired Pneumonia in Children. *Pediatrics*, Feb 2005; 115: 517.
14. Reed W., Byrd G., Gates R., Howard R., Weaver, M.; Sputum Gram's Stain in Community-acquired *Pneumococcal* Pneumonia: a Meta-analysis. *Western Journal of Medicine.* 1996;165(4):197-204.
15. Tsutomu Yamazaki, Kei Murayama, Atsuko Ito, Suzuko Uehara, and Nozomu Sasaki. Epidemiology of Community-Acquired Pneumonia in Children. *Pediatrics*, Feb 2005; 115: 517.
16. Wilmott, R., Kaplan, E., Perez, C., Hardi.e., W, Chini, B., Daines, C.; *Pediatric Secrets*, 3rd Ed. Ch 18; pp 664-668.
17. Viessman, S., Lorin, M.; *Appleton & Lange Review of Pediatrics: Infectious Disease.* Ch 7 p 132, 144.

Rapid Sequence Intubation (RSI)

Frederick Bartoletti, MD
Department of Emergency Medicine
The University of Arizona

Critical Knowledge

- Survival after cardiac arrest in children averages 7% to 11%, with most survivors neurologically impaired. For this reason early recognition and treatment of respiratory failure and shock is essential to prevent an arrest from occurring.
- Indications for intubation
  - Respiratory failure
  - Inadequate ventilation or inadequate oxygenation
  - Anticipated respiratory failure
  - Airway protection
  - Anticipated airway obstruction

Antipate Respiratory Failure Signs

- An increased respiratory rate, particularly with signs of distress (e.g., increased effort, nasal flaring, retractions, or grunting)
- An inadequate respiratory rate, effort, or chest excursion (e.g., diminished breath sounds, gasping, and cyanosis)
- Depressed mental status in the presence of abnormal respiration

Indicators of Difficult Airway

- Inability to extend neck beyond 35 degrees
- Thyromental distance greater that 2 adult fingerwidths (3 cm) from the ramus to the thyroid cartilage in adolescent or child, or more than one fingerwidth in infants
- Limited mandible motion (i.e., JRA, scoliosis, trismus, facial fractures)
- Congenital anomalies. Cleft palate, micrognathia, macroglossia, glossoptosis, maxillary or mandibular anomalies, protruding maxillary incisors.
- Airway obstruction. Bleeding, infection, burns, cervical fractures, inhalation injury, foreign body.

Rapid Sequence Intubation

- To facilitate emergency intubation and reduce the incidence of complications
- Sedatives, neuromuscular blocking agents, and other medications rapidly sedate and paralyze the patient
- Used by trained and experienced providers in evaluation and management of the pediatric airway.
- If you use RSI you must have a secondary plan to manage the airway in the event that you cannot achieve intubation.
- Cuffed versus uncuffed tubes
- In the in-hospital setting a cuffed endotracheal tube is as safe as an uncuffed tube for infants beyond the newborn period and in children.[1]
- In certain circumstances (e.g., poor lung compliance, high airway resistance, or a large glottic air leak) a cuffed tube may be preferable provided that attention is paid to endotracheal tube size, position, and cuff inflation pressure.[1]
- Keep cuff inflation pressure <20 cm H_2O.

Helpful pediatric formulas

- Weight (kg) = (2 * age in years) + 8
- ETT size (mm) = (age in years + 16)/4
- ETT placement at lip = 3 * normal estimated tube size
- Drugs that can be given through ETT
- **NAVEL** (***N****arcan*, ***A****tropine*, ***V****alium*, ***E****pinephrine*, ***L****idocaine*)
- Background/Epidemiology/Anatomy
- Airway compromise is the most common cause of cardiac arrest death and severe morbidity in acutely ill and injured children.

Adverse Effects of Intubation

- **I**ntra**C**ranial **P**ressure (**ICP**) increases (theoretical)
- Airway trauma
- Pain
- Bradycardia
- Tachycardia
- Gastric regurgitation
- Aspiration

- Hypoxemia
- Arrhythmias
- Death

Anatomy

- Proportionally larger head and occiput cause neck flexion and airway obstruction when the child is supine
- Larger tongue results in less oral space
- Decreased muscle tone causes passive airway obstruction by the tongue
- The epiglottis is shorter, narrower, more horizontal, and softer
- The larynx is more anterior, making visualization of the cords more difficult
- The trachea is shorter increasing the risk of right main stem intubation
- The airway is narrower increasing airway resistance
- The cricoid ring is the narrowest portion of the airway

Differential Diagnosis/Critical Concepts

- Infection
- Trauma
- Decreased GCS (<8)
- Chest trauma
- Neck trauma
- Burns
- Foreign body
- CHF
- Asthma
- Respiratory arrest

Treatment

- Adjuncts for maintaining an open airway
- Oropharyngeal and nasopharyngeal airways
    - ▸ Oropharyngeal airways are used in unconscious victims (i.e., with no gag reflex). Select the correct size: an oropharyngeal airway that is too small will not keep the tongue from obstructing the pharynx; one that is too large may obstruct the airway. Correctly sized airway will extend from the patient's mouth to the angle of the jaw. Not tolerated in patients with a gag response.

- Nasopharyngeal airways: better tolerated than oral airways by patients who are not deeply unconscious. Small nasopharyngeal tubes (for infants) may be easily obstructed by secretions. Correctly sized airway will extend from the nare to the tragus. Should be inserted perpendicularly to the face.

- Laryngeal mask airway: there is insufficient evidence to recommend for or against the routine use of a **L**aryngeal **L**ask **A**irway (**LMA**) during cardiac arrest. When endotracheal intubation is not possible, the LMA is an acceptable adjunct for experienced providers, but it is associated with a higher incidence of complications in young children.[2]

RSI Pretreatment

- **MAIDS**: (**M**onitor, **A**irway equipment, **I**V, **D**rugs, **S**uction)
- A bunch of P's: preoxygenate, prepare equipment, position patient, premedicate, push sedative, push on cricoid, paralyze, place tube, confirm position
- Premedication
  - **LOAD**
    - ***L**idocaine* (1.5 mg/kg) mixed evidence on transient decrease in ICP and intraocular pressure
    - ***O**piate* (*fentanyl* 2-3 mcg/kg IV) sympatholytic theoretically lessens ICP
    - ***A**tropine* (0.02 mg/kg IV minimum dose 0.1mg, maximum 1mg) indicated if age <5 when using *succinylcholine*, or when bradycardic prior to intubation.
    - **D**efasciculating dose (one tenth the paralytic dose)
  - RSI induction
    - *Etomodate* (0.3 mg/kg IV) not FDA approved for <10 years old
    - *Ketamine* (0.5-2 mg/kg IV) preferred in presence of bronchospasm, avoid if elevated ICP
    - *Thiopental* (3-5 mg/kg IV) preferred if suspected elevated ICP, use half dose in presence of hypotension
    - *Versed* (0.1-0.2 mg/kg) lowers BP, HR, RR
    - Apply cricoid pressure immediately after giving induction agent

- RSI paralysis
    - *Succinylcholine* (1-2 mg/kg IV) pretreat with *atropine* if <5 years old for first and all subsequent doses, avoid if suspected hyperkalemia, neuromuscular disorder, muscular dystrophy, family history of malignant hyperthermia
    - Pretreat with a nondepolarizing agent
    - *Rocuronium* (0.6-1.2 mg/kg IV) onset one minute, lasts 30 minutes

Tube Placement

- Cricoid pressure should be placed after induction
- Avoid BVM ventilation to prevent gastric insufflation, helping to prevent emesis
- Tube confirmation
    - There is a high risk that an endotracheal tube will be misplaced (i.e., placed in the esophagus or in the pharynx above the vocal chords), displaced, or become obstructed, especially when the patient is moved, or mainstemed.
    - No single confirmation technique is completely reliable, so providers must use both clinical assessment and confirmatory devices to verify proper tube placement.
    - Confirmation of correct tube position must be completed immediately after intubation and again after securing the tube, or any time you move the patient.
    - Bilateral chest movement and equal breath sounds over both lung fields, especially over the axillae.
    - Listen for gastric insufflation sounds over the stomach (they should not be present if the tube is in the trachea).
    - CO_2 detector if there is a perfusing rhythm.
    - If the child has a perfusing rhythm and is >20 kg, you may use an esophageal detector device to check for evidence of esophageal placement.
    - Check oxygen saturation with a pulse oximeter. Following hyperoxygenation, the oxyhemoglobin saturation detected by pulse oximetry may not demonstrate a fall indicative of incorrect endotracheal tube position (i.e., tube misplacement or displacement) for as long as 3 minutes.

    - If you are still uncertain, perform direct laryngoscopy and look to see if the tube goes between the cords.
    - In the hospital settings perform a chest x-ray to verify that the tube is not in the right main bronchus and to identify a high tube position at risk of easy displacement.
- Secure the tube
    - There is insufficient evidence to recommend any one method. After you secure the tube
    - Maintain the patient's head in a neutral position
    - Neck flexion pushes the tube farther into the airway
    - Neck extension pulls the tube out of the airway
- Failed Airway
    - LMA insertion
    - Cricothyroidotomy is of value in severe facial trauma
    - Contraindicated if less than 8 years old
    - Needle cricothyroidotomy with transtracheal jet ventilation
    - Digital tracheal intubation
    - Retrograde endotracheal intubation

Trouble Shooting an Intubated/Ventilated Patient

- DOPE
    - Displacement of the tube from the trachea
    - Obstruction of the tube
    - Pneumothorax

Questions

1. A 5 year old boy is the victim of a near drowning accident. Paramedics started CPR in the field and the child's ventilation was assisted with BVM. On arrival to the ED the child has cardiac activity and pulses. What size endotracheal tube should you use on this child?

    A. 4

    B. 4.5

    C. 5

    D. 5.5

    Answer: C

2. An 18 month old child is suffering from respiratory failure in the ED from RSV. Upon evaluation for securing an airway for ventilation you notice that the patient's vitals are HR 95, BP 80/40, RR 70, Temp 38.4. What pretreatment with the correct dose do you want to give this child?
   A. *Lidocaine* 1.5 mg/kg
   B. *Atropine* 0.02 mg/kg
   C. *Lidocaine* 0.02 mg/kg
   D. *Atropine* 1.5 mg/kg

   Answer: B
3. Which of the following alternative airway techniques would not be indicated for a 4 year old after failing at RSI endotracheal intubation?
   A. LMA
   B. Cricothyroidotomy
   C. BVM
   D. Transtracheal jet ventilation

   Answers: B

References

1. Newth CJ, Rachman B, Patel N, Hammer J. The use of cuffed versus uncuffed endotracheal tubes in pediatric intensive care. *J Pediatr.* 2004;144 :333 –337
2. Berry AM, Brimacombe JR, Verghese C. The laryngeal mask airway in emergency medicine, neonatal resuscitation, and intensive care medicine. *Int Anesthesiol Clin.* 1998;36:91–109.
3. 2005 AHA Guidelines for Cardiopulmonary Resuscitation and Emergency Cardiovascular Care. Part 12: Pediatric Advanced Life Support. *Circulation* 2005:112/IV-167-VI-187
4. Gerardi M J, Sacchetti AD, Cantor RM, Santamaria JP, Gausche M, Lucid W, Foltin GL: Rapid-sequence intubation of the pediatric patient. *Ann Emerg Med July* 1996;28:55-74.
5. Moynihan RJ, Brock-Utne JG, Archer JH, Feld LH, Kreitzman TR. The effect of cricoid pressure on preventing gastric insufflation in infants and children. *Anesthesiology.* 1993; 78: 652–656

Sedation

Lisa Doyle, MD
Attending Physician
Utah Emergency Physicians

Critical Knowledge

- Only a provider who is skilled in pediatric resuscitation and management of the pediatric airway should perform pediatric sedation.
- This provider must have an understanding of the serious side effects of the medications.
- Know your goal: sedation, analgesia, or both.
- Pulse oximetry is not useful in the detection of hypoventilation when using supplemental oxygen. Monitoring the patient's chest rise and the measurement of exhaled carbon dioxide are more reliable.

Background

Procedural sedation is safe, effective, and humane way to facilitate appropriate medical care. Analgesics and sedatives can be used alone or together to achieve the desired effect. Use the combination of an analgesic with a sedative for painful procedures. Use a sedative alone for painless unpleasant procedures (i.e., MRI). Keep in mind that the opioid analgesics will also provide sedation at high dosages, but using these dosages will also increase the risk of unwanted side effects such as respiratory depression.

Medications for Sedation and Analgesia		
Medications	**Contraindications**	**Negative effects**
Opioid Analgesics		
Morphine		Respiratory depression, hypotension, nausea, pruritis
Fentanyl		Respiratory depression, hypotension, nausea, nasal pruritis
Meperidine	Concurrent use with SSRI or MAOI	Lowers seizure threshold, hypotention, long half-life
Benzodiazepine		
Midazolam	Hypotension or the potential for cardiovascular collapse	Respiratory depression, hypotension, disinhibition with paradoxical excitement

Barbiturates		
Methohexital	Age <3 years	Hypotension, respiratory depression
Pentobarbital	Liver failure, hyperactivity, age >8 years	Irritability, hyperactivity, nausea
Alkyl Phenol		
Propofol	Egg or soy allergy, hypotension or the potential for cardiovascular collapse	Pain at injection site, hypo/ hypertension, apnea
Dissociative Agent		
Ketamine	Age <3 months, psychosis, elevated ICP, seizures, active asthma, porphyria, thyroid disease	Unpleasant emergent reactions, laryngospasm, increased secretions*, nausea *May use *atropine* 0.01-0.2 mg/kg IV to reduce secretions
Hypnotic		
Etomidate	Seizure disorder, age <12 years	Myoclonus, pain at injection site
Antihistamine		
Diphenhydramine	Neonates, premature infants, non-reversible—do not use if you need to follow neurological status	Hallucination in overdose
Sedative Hypnotic		
Chloral Hydrate	Nonreversible—do not use if you need to follow neurological status	Erratic mucosal absorption, paradoxical excitement
Opioid Antagonist		
Naloxone		
***Benzodiazepine* Antagonist**		
Flumazenil	*Benzodiazepine* use >2weeks, increased ICP	

Medication Properties		
Analgesics	**Sedatives/Anxiolytics**	**Analgesia+ Sedation**
Morphine	*Midazolam*	*Ketamine*
Fentanyl	*Methohexital*	
Meperidine	*Pentobarbital*	
	Propofol	
	Etomidate	
	Chloral Hydrate	
	Diphenhydramine	

Duration of Action		
Drug	**Route**	**Duration**
Morphine	IV	3-5 hours
	IM	3-5 hours
Fentanyl	IV	20-30 min
Meperidine	IV	3-4 hours
Midazolam	IV	20-30 min
	IM	1-2 hours
	IN	1 hour
	PO	1-1.5 hours
	PR	30-60 min
Methohexital	IV	10 min
	PR	45 min
Pentobarbital	IV	15-45 min
	IM	1-2 hours
	PO/PR	1-4 hours
Propofol	IV	5-10 min
Ketamine	IV	5-10 min
	IM	20-30 min
Etomidate	IV	20 min
Diphenhydramine	IV	2-6 hours
	PO	4-6 hours
Chloral Hydrate	PO/PR	1-2 hours
Nalaxone	IV	15-30 min
	IM	1-1.5 hours
Flumazenil	IV	20-60 min

Treatment

When performing a procedure requiring sedation in the ED, one provider must be dedicated solely to the aspect of sedation.

- A suggested checklist for the essentials of sedation
  - Pre-sedation history and physical
  - Pre-sedation vital signs
  - PALS resuscitation equipment
  - Age appropriate airway equipment
  - Continuous cardiac monitoring, non-invasive BP, end tidal CO2 monitoring
  - Supplemental oxygen
  - Ability to obtain rapid IV access if using IM sedation
- During the sedation vital signs should be monitored continuously
- The most dangerous part of the sedation is AFTER the procedure when the noxious stimulus is over. This is the time when respiratory depression will most likely occur.
- A child should not be discharged home until the following conditions are met
  - Protecting own airway
  - Returned to baseline mental and ambulatory status
  - Pain is well controlled

Questions

1. A 2 year old child arrives in your emergency department after a head injury. She has a boggy right parietal scalp hematoma and needs a brain CT. She is sleepy with purposeful movements and is inconsolable. What are good options for sedation for the CT?

   A. *Midazolam*

   B. *Propofol*

   C. *Ketamine*

   D. *Etomidate*

   E. A or B

   Answer: E; Both *midazolam* and *propofol* could be good choices. Keep in mind that *Propofol* has the potential for significant respiratory depression. This child will need close monitoring while in the radiology department.

2. A 13 year old asthmatic child arrives at 6pm with a significantly angulated distal radius fracture. She needs her fracture reduced. She had "some water" at soccer practice 2 hours ago, and last ate solids "at lunch at school." She has no allergies, and only uses her albuterol inhaler about once a month when she exercises outside. Is she a good candidate for procedural sedation for her fracture reduction?
   A. No! She needs to be NPO for at least 8 hours
   B. No! She is an asthmatic
   C. Yes! She meets the ASA NPO guidelines for a safe sedation
   D. Yes! She is an ASA class II, with a mild systemic disease that is well controlled on medications
   E. C and D

   Answer: E; It is safe to perform procedural sedation on this patient. ASA physical status of 3-4 are considered high risk for sedation by the non-anesthesiologist.

3. An 8 year old healthy male arrives with extensive road-rash, multiple lacerations, and embedded gravel after a scooter crash. These are his only injuries. He requires debridement, foreign body removal, and laceration repairs. He weighs 30 kg. What is the best way to proceed?
   A. Scrub away, haven't you heard of "brutane?"
   B. Apply copious amounts of viscous *lidocaine* to the roadrash, an inject the lacerations and foreign bodies with as much local *lidocaine* as needed to achicvc analgcsia.
   C. Use *ketamine* as a dissociative anesthetic or a combination of an opioid analgesic and a sedative.
   D. Use procedural sedation along with distraction techniques and adjunct local analgesia.
   E. C or D

   Answer: E; "Brutane," or the use of brut force to just hold a child during painful procedures is not appropriate in this situation. Topical and injected *lidocaines* are great adjuncts for pain relief, but you need to be careful to consider the maximum dosage especially in a small child with extensive injuries.

References

1. Godwin S, Caro D, Wolf S, et al. Clinical policy for procedural sedation and analgesia in the emergency department. *Ann Emerg Med* 2005;45:177-96
2. American Society of Anesthesiologists. Practice guidelines for sedation and analgesia by non-anesthesiologists: an updated report by the American Society of Anesthesiologists Task Force on Sedation and Analgesia by Non-Anesthesiologists. *Anesthesiology* 2002;96:1004-17

Sport Specific Injury

Becky Doran, MD
Assistant Professor of Emergency Medicine and Pediatrics
Department of Emergency Medicine and Pediatrics
Indiana University School of Medicine

Critical Concepts

- Individual sports are highly associated with specific injury patterns
- Recognize and address acute issues of specific sports
- Recognize the signs and symptoms of concussion and refer for long term care
- Re-injury syndrome following closed head injury can have devastating consequences
- Be a true advocate for the child by exercising caution when giving permission for return-to-play

Introduction

Sports injuries are one of the most common reasons pediatric patients will be brought to the emergency department. As an emergency physician it is important to be cognizant of the common injuries associated with a particular sport and with the high risk injuries that can lead to poor outcomes. (Table 1)

Child athletes have different injury mechanisms, types and distribution than their adult counterparts. An understanding of this can help the emergency medicine physician guide treatment and address the unique concerns of the child athlete and their parents.

Table: 1	
Sport	**Common Injuries**
Baseball	'Little league elbow'/ shoulder injuries
Basketball	Hand fractures/dislocations Knee injuries
Bicycling	Head injury Genitourinary injury
Boxing	Fifth metacarpal fracture Eye injury
Dancing	Base of fifth metatarsal fracture

Sport	Common Injuries
Diving	Spinal cord injury
Football	Concussion/C-spine injury ACL tears
Golf	Elbow injury
Gymnastics	Back fractures
Hockey	Intracranial injury
Horseback Riding	C-spine/back fractures Shoulder injury
Ice Skating	Ankle injury
Running	Lower extremity stress fractures Heat injury
Soccer	ACL Tear
Swimming	Rotator cuff injury
Tennis	Elbow injury
Wrestling	Rotator cuff injury Lower extremity ligamentous injury

Concussion

Critical Knowledge

Consussion is a common injury in adolescent contact sports. Often the signs of a concussion are not obvious and can easily be mistaken for other processes by emergency physicians. Return to play is the ever present question from parents, athletes and coaches and a firm and educated response is required. Second impact or re-injury syndrome is a real threat to those athletes that have had a prior injury.

Background

- *Definition:* A concussion is an injury to the brain that results in temporary loss of normal brain function.[1]
- A concussion does not always include a loss of consciousness.
- 15-20% of high school football players will receive a concussion during a single season.[1]
- Emergency physicians will be approached for advice or permission regarding the athlete's ability to return to play. (Table 2)

Symptoms of a Concussion	
Prolonged headache	Balance impairment
Vision disturbance	Difficulty concentrating
Memory loss	Sensitivity to light
Irritability	Ringing in ears
Sleep disturbance	Loss of smell or taste
Nausea or vomiting	Dizziness

Diagnostics

- Complete neurologic exam
  - Cranial nerves
  - Cerebellar exam
  - Strength testing
- Visual acuity exam
- Head CT, if warranted
  - Loss of consciousness
  - Abnormal exam
  - Persistent symptoms

Treatment/Disposition

- Neurosurgery consultation for any abnormal head CT
- Symptomatic treatment for headache, nausea, etc.
- Close follow up with primary care provider for repeat exams and return to play advice
- Potential follow up with neurology or neuropsych testing if persistent symptoms

Second Impact Syndrome

Critical Knowledge

An uncommon but devastating injury is reported in those athletes who have sustained a prior concussion and suffer a "second hit." The lifetime accumulation of concussion, brain injury, leads to long term effects. Athletes that have had one concussion prior are much more likely to suffer a second than those who have never had a head injury.

Background

- Risk of concussion is **6 times** more likely in a player who has previously suffered a concussion.
- Second impact syndrome is reported in the literature and is thought to have caused several instances of athlete sudden death on the playing field.
- After a brain injury the brain needs recovery time and a second injury during that recovery period can lead to irreversible damage.

Treatment/Disposition

- Emergent airway management and immediate consultation with neurosurgery for ICP monitoring
- Evaluation with head CT and MRI for injury assessment
- If recovery, restriction from contact sports completely

Return to Play

Critical Concepts

Knowledge of return to play guidelines' is critical for the emergency physician. Parents, coaches and athletes want to return as soon as possible, often with compelling reasons (scholarships, etc.). A working understanding of guidelines and educational approach for families will best protect young athletes from re-injury.

Background

- There is no consensus statement from the societies on return to play.
- The Cantu guidelines are the most conservative and one of the most widely used. (Table 2)

Treatment

- Follow up with primary care physician before return to play is always indicatied for young athletes to ensure the the sublte signs of continued brain recovery are not missed.
- Setting up an athlete and families expectations for return to play with the most conservative guidelines is recommended.

Table 2: Cantu Return to Play Guidelines[3]		
Grade	**Definition**	**Return to Play**
Grade I	No loss of consciousness No persistent amnesia (must last less than 30 minutes)	When completely symptom free for seven days
Grade II	Brief loss of consciousness (less than 5 minutes) – or memory loss between 30 minutes and 24 hours	When completely symptom free for seven days For repeat concussion sidelined for season
Grade III	Loss of consciousness for more than 5 minutes – or memory loss for greater than 24 hours duration	Out of play for one month, then may return to play only if symptom free for seven consecutive days after the restricted month

Questions

1. A fifteen year old male football player presents to the emergency department with a persistent headache after a tackle in his weekend game 4 days prior. He also complains of trouble sleeping and concentrating in school over the past few days. His neurologic exam is normal. What is your recommendation on the big district game this weekend (three days away)?
   A. Head CT; if negative allow play
   B. Head CT; if negative and headache gone by game allow play
   C. Tylenol and continue to monitor, have school trainer reexamine prior to game, if no focal neurologic findings allow play
   D. Do not allow play in the weekend game; must be completely symptom free for 7 days prior to any resumed contact activity
   E. Suspend play for the season

   Answer: D

References

1. American Association of Neurological Surgeons. www.neurosurgerytoday.org.
2. Collins et al., Current Issues in Managing Sports-Related Concussion, *JAMA*.1999; 282: 2283-2285.
3. Cantu, Robert. Cantu Guidelines.

Ligamentous Injury and Dislocations

Critical Concepts

Although becoming more common in the adolescent ages (ACL tears), in general ligamentous injury and dislocations in isolation are relatively uncommon in the pediatric population. An astute emergency physician will search for the hidden fracture or other injury in a young child who at first glance appears to have only a ligamentous injury or dislocation.

Background

- Ligamentous injury and in there most severe form, dislocations, are uncommon in very young children and generally are associated with fractures.
- Ligaments in children are much more elastic and stronger than boney structures.[1]
- Subluxation of the radial head in toddlers, or "nursemaids elbow" is the one exception to this general principle.
  - *Subluxation of radial head*
    - Exam: arm held pronated and extended (limp by child's side). Child is not distressed until limb is moved.
    - If signs and symptoms are typical of nursemaids elbow a radiograph is not mandatory. If the history is atypical or there is focal swelling a radiograph should be done to exclude supracondylar or radial head fracture.
    - Treat by holding child's hand and with the other hand encircle the elbow, thumb over radial head. Apply traction and supinate the hand while flexing the forearm at the elbow. You should feel a pop as the radial head is relocated. The child should move the arm normally within 30 minutes.

Treatment

- Pain control
- Stabilization of the injury with splinting in functional position
- Close follow up in consultation with orthopaedic surgery
- Joint dislocations from injury are emergent because they can be associated with arterial injury which places the entire distal limb at risk. Most are managed with immediate closed reduction. These patients should receive

urgent follow up as some of these injuries in young athletes (shoulder dislocations, ACL tears) do very poorly with conservative treatment and usually require surgical intervention.

Questions

1. A 2 year old child is brought in after her parents noted that she would not use her right arm at dinner. They were at the zoo during the day and had been swinging her through the parking lot on the way to the car, at the time she had complained of the arm but fallen asleep in the car seat and "seemed okay." She is now in no distress with her right arm hanging limply at her side; no external signs of injury/swelling are present. What should your plan be?
   A. X-ray then reduction of subluxed radial head
   B. Immediate reduction of subluxed radial head with a post reduction observation period for function return
   C. X-ray of the entire arm and consultation with orthopedics
   D. Splinting of the arm after X-ray and follow up in one week as an outpatient
   E. IV pain medication, conscious sedation and closed reduction
   Answer: B

References

1. *Pediatrics in Review.* 2000;21:433-434.
2. *http://www.emedicine.com*

Fractures

Critical Concepts

A fracture should be suspected in any child presenting with deformity, swelling or localized boney tenderness of a limb after an injury. In very young children not moving the limb or weight bearing refusal may be indicative of the injury. Fractures in children follow a different injury pattern due to the growth plate and the relative strength imbalance between the growth areas and ligaments.

Background

- Salter Harris fractures common
- Greenstick and Buckle fractures in young children
- May be missed in acute injury period, if still suspicious repeat x-rays in 5-7 days

Salter–Harris Classification of Epiphyseal Injuries	
Fracture Type	**Description**
Salter-Harris I	Slipped growth plate
Salter- Harris II	Fracture through metaphysis
Salter- Harris III	Fracture through epiphysis
Salter- Harris IV	Fracture through epiphysis and metaphysis
Salter- Harris V	Crush or compression of growth plate

Diagnostics

- An x-ray should be obtained of any suspected fracture site and should often include the joints on either side.
- Comparison views of the contralateral side should NOT be done routinely, but on occasion may be helpful in interpretation (elbow).

Treatment

- Fractures are painful and effective splinting early along with adequate pain medication can greatly improve the patients' outlook.
- If fracture is not immediately apparent but mechanism and suspicion is high, splinting and repeat films in 5-7 days is recommended to rule out an occult fracture.
- Fracture follow up should include referral to an orthopedist for further management and repeat imaging after one week to ensure proper alignment of fracture area.

References

1. Young, Simon et al. *MJA* 2005; 182 (12:644-648.

Sprains and Strains

Critical Knowledge

Sprains and strains do occur in the young athlete and may indicate over use of a particular muscle group. These injuries should be considered a diagnosis of exclusion in the younger age group because a disproportionate number of children complaining of painful areas after a sports injury will have a fracture.

Background

- SPRAIN – overstretching and stress to a ligament
- Sprains are most common in sports with a high frequency of twisting/ cutting movements.
- Sprains are more common in adolescent athletes and do not tend to occur in younger children because the epiphyseal plates are the weak link in an injury event and are more likely to fracture.
- STRAIN- damage to the muscle, as a result of forceful contraction.
- Children and adolescents who have recently gone through a growth spurt are at higher risk of suffering from strains.
- The most common sites for strains to occur are in the hamstrings, quadriceps and the calf muscles.[1]

Treatment

- Management of the mild to moderate sprain (fracture excluded) should follow the **RICE** pneumonic
  - **R**est: minimal weight bearing until acute pain subsides then encourage mobilization and range of motion exercise.
  - **I**ce: applied every 4 hours for 15 minutes over the first 48 hours
  - **C**ompression: firm bandaging for 48 hours only
  - **E**levations: elevate whenever possible to allow swelling to subside
- Severe sprain or strains may benefit from physical therapy as part of rehabilitation.
- Follow up should be ensured for all of these children from the emergency department to a primary physician who can assess progress and make rehabilitation decisions.

Heat Stress Injury

Critical Knowledge

Heat injuries include heat cramps, heat exhaustion and heat stroke which is a life threatening emergency. These injuries must be recognized early and immediately treated to prevent complications. Education for the parents and coaches of children athletes is crucial in reducing this injury.

Background

- Children acclimate to heat more slowly than adults because of less heat dissipation and a lower sweat rate.
- Children can adjust to temperatures with proper clothing (breathable), hydration (frequent breaks) and proper monitoring.
- If any signs of heat emergency are present the child should be brought to medical attention and cooling should begin immediately.

Treatment

- Protect airway, breathing circulation in critical patients and respond appropriately
- Assess core temperature
- Begin immediate cooling measures to include remove all clothing, cooling blankets, cold water, baths, etc.
- Rehydration
- Restriction from activities following a heat emergency and close follow up with a primary physician that can follow and educate.

References

1. Hutchinson, Mark, *Common Sports Injuries in Children and Adolescents.* 19 July 2000.

The Crying Infant

Brian D. Clothier, MD, MS
Instructor, Division of Emergency Medicine
Attending Physician, Emergency Department, Primary Children's Medical Center
University of Utah

Critical Concept

Evaluation of the fussy or crying infant requires a certain amount of finesse. Paroxysms of crying are common in the second to third week of life and many bewildered parents will present seeking reassurance. However, many serious or even life-threatening diseases will present during the infant period as crying and inconsolability.

Quick tips

- **Take a complete history**. In the newborn period, this should include a prenatal history including maternal gravity and parity, prenatal care, and infection risks. The birth history should include gestational age and weight and complications of pregnancy and delivery. The nature and onset of the crying as well as associated symptoms are particularly important. This information will help you determine if the infant is at risk for infection, congenital anomaly, abuse or neglect.
- **All fussy infants are presumed ill until proven otherwise**. Most are not critically ill, but to presume the worst will force you to be thorough in your history, physical examination and thought process.
- **Use time to your advantage**. Consider observing the patient in the ED over several hours. It is easier to make subtle diagnoses when the patient is re-examined over time and will provide you and the parent reassurance of a benign diagnosis. Benign causes of crying will cease eventually.

Background

Infants and children presenting with "crying" or "fussiness" are extremely common. Parents may describe these children as "just not acting right." Etiologies range from benign to life-threatening. As always in medicine, a broad differential is the key to making the correct diagnosis.

Remember

- **Establish the pattern of crying, exacerbating factors, and other signs of illness.** Parents will define "fussy" differently based on their frame of reference which varies based on their culture, socioeconomic status, and parenting experience.

- **Benign etiologies are diagnoses of exclusion!**
- **Consider child abuse.** Any sign of trauma in an infant must raise your suspicion of abuse. Consider also the abuse you may prevent by identifying at-risk situations.
- **5% will have multiple causes of their illness, whatever it may be.**

Differential Diagnosis

The single most important action in the evaluation of the fussy infant is to build an appropriate differential diagnosis and then, either by history, physical exam, or testing, rule out each diagnosis. The following table contains some more common causes of infant fussiness.

Conditions Associated with Crying or Fussy Infants and Young Children - Adapted from Fleisher	
Head and Neck	• Encephalitis/meningitis • Skull fracture/subdural hematoma • Glaucoma • Eye foreign body/corneal abrasion • Acute otitis media • Pseudotumor cerebri
Respiratory	• Upper respiratory infections • Viral prodromes: myalgia/arthralgia
Cardiovascular	• Coarctation of the aorta • Congestive heart failure • SVT • Anomalous origin of left coronary artery from pulmonary artery
Gastrointestinal	• Gastroesophageal reflux/esophagitis • Gastritis/gastroenteritis • Appendicitis • Intussusception • Volvulus • Cow's milk protein intolerance • Excess gastrointestinal air • Anal fissure

Genitourinary	• Testicular torsion • Incarcerated hernia • UTI
Integumentary	• Burn • Strangulated finger, toe, penis (hair tourniquet)
Toxic/ Metabolic	• Drugs: *antihistamines, atropinics, adrenergics, cocaine* (including passive inhalation), *aspirin* • Toxic ingestions/ overdose • Metabolic acidosis, hypernatremia, hypocalcemia, hypoglycemia
Musculoskeletal	• Extremity fracture from fall or child abuse
Trauma	• Falls • Physical abuse/neglect
Behavioral	• Colic • Parental anxiety

Treatment Strategy

For all crying or fussy children, a systematic approach to the history and physical will lead you in the right direction.

- **Observe the interaction between the parent and child.** A child who will not console even momentarily while eating or sleeping is potentially ill.
- **Physical examination.** Scrutinize the vital signs, including HR and BP. Thorough physical evaluation includes examination of the corneas and retinas, otoscopy with pneumatic insufflation, auscultation of heart and lungs, palpation of abdomen, palpation of long bones, genital exam, anal exam with/without rectal exam and complete skin exam for bruising or other lesions. Examine the extremities, including the penis, for signs of trauma, hair tourniquet, and perfusion.
- **Take off the diaper.** Critical diagnoses such as anal fissure, testicular torsion, hair-tourniquet, inguinal hernia or intussusception will be missed without this key portion of the physical exam.
- **There is no "fussy infant" work up.** Order lab work, imaging studies and consultation based on your thorough history and physical examination.
- **It is dangerous to discharge a child who is not consolable and for whom you do not have a firm diagnosis.**

Pearls for Specific Pathologies not Covered Elsewhere in this Text

- **Pseudotumor Cerebri:** consider this diagnosis in a crying infant with a bulging fontanelle in whom you have ruled out intracranial infection, mass, bleeding, and hydrocephalus. Opening pressure at lumbar puncture will be elevated.
- **Corneal Abrasion:** Look for a unilateral red eye without discharge in an otherwise well-appearing infant. Make certain to flouricine stain the eyes of any crying infant with unknown etiology.
- **Supraventricular Tachycardia (SVT):** Obtain an ECG on any infant with a heart rate greater than 200 bpm. SVT in infants will have a rate >220. The history will be incompatible with sinus tachycardia, p waves will be absent and the heart rate may change dramatically. Hemodynamically unstable infants should be cardioverted.
- **Anal Fissure:** More common at ages when infants transition to solid foods (4-6 months), cow's milk (12 months) or associated with toilet training. History will describe hard, bowel movements associated with straining. The diagnosis can often be made by history before confirmation of fissure on physical exam.

References

1. Pawel BB, Henretig FM, Crying and Colic in Early Infancy. In: Fleisher GR, Ludwig S, eds. Textbook of *Pediatric Emergency Medicine, 4th Ed.* Philadelphia, PA: Lippencott Williams & Wilkins; 2000: 193-195.

Colic

Brian D. Clothier, MD, MS
Instructor, Division of Emergency Medicine
Attending Physician, Emergency Department, Primary Children's Medical Center
University of Utah

Critical Knowledge

Colic is Defined by the Rule of 3s

- Crying more than three hours per day, for more than three days per week, and for more than three weeks in an infant that is well-fed and otherwise healthy.[1]
- Colic is a diagnosis of exclusion! Always consider life-threatening diagnoses first!

Background

- Symptoms begin as early as two weeks of age and usually resolve by 4 months
- Symptoms tend to occur in the late afternoon or early evening
- As the name implies, colic is considered to be abdominal pain related to the colon
- The symptoms vary but can include high-pitched cries, grimaces, knees pulled to chest
- By definition, the colicky infant is difficult to console and as such can be very stressful to inexperienced or overwhelmed parents

Differential Diagnosis

Any of the conditions listed in table (see page 276) can cause abrupt onset of crying in a young infant and should be considered and ruled out prior to diagnosing colic.

Key Concepts

- Ascertain the length and frequency of crying as well as associated signs and symptoms.
- A thorough physical examination is paramount and should include gastrointestinal and neurological examination.
- Radiographic imaging and lab studies are unnecessary in an otherwise healthy-appearing infant.[2]

Treatment

Various strategies exist for managing colic, but there are few evidence-based guidelines.

Diet

- No evidence exists for changing the diet.
- Breast-feeding mothers must be encouraged to continue nurse.
- Infants taking cow milk-based formulas should only be switched to hypoallergenic formulas such as casein or whey hydrolysate if there is suspicion for milk-protein allergy as evidenced by loose-bloody stools or other signs of atopy (rhinitis, wheezing, atopic dermatitis) or a family history of atopy. 30% of children with cow-milk protein allergy will also be allergic to soy protein; therefore switching to soy formula is without basis and is not recommended in the management of colic.[3]

Medications

- Anticholinergics have been described to aid in resolution of colic.[4] However, they are also rarely associated with apnea, seizures, and syncope and as such cannot be recommended. *Dicyclomine* (*Bentyl*) should be avoided in children younger than six months because of an association with apnea.
- Simethicone drops are purported to break up gas bubbles but have not been shown more effective than placebo.[5]
- Various herbal remedies are widely available without prescription. Some may be helpful in the treatment of colic. There are no randomized, controlled trials of these products and as such, parents should be educated and cautioned about their use.

Behavioral Modifications

- Taking the infant for a ride in the car is near-universally believed to help with colic but is an unproven technique.
- Evidence does not support expensive and potentially dangerous interventions including car-ride simulators, crib vibrators and buckling the infant in a car seat placed atop a running clothes dryer.[1]
- Parents should be taught techniques to soothe the baby including the 4 **S**'s: **S**hushing (white noise), **S**waddling (simulates intrauterine environment), **S**winging (produces soothing motion), and **S**ucking (on a breast or pacifier).

Questions

1. What is the Rule of 3's for colic?

   Answer: 1) Crying more than three hours per day, 2) for more than three days per week, and 3) more than three weeks in an infant that is well-fed and otherwise healthy.

2. Which of the following is NOT one of the rules in the "Rule of 3's" for colic?

   A. Three o'clock in the morning

   B. Three hours a day

   C. Three days a week

   D. Three weeks long

   Answer: A

3. When should the diet of a colicky infant be changed?

   A. Never

   B. To appease the parents so they feel something is being done.

   C. When there is evidence of a mild protein allergy

   D. Excessive gas noted by parents

   Answer: C

4. Which medication has been proven safe and effective in the treatment of colic?

   A. *Dicyclomine* (*bentyl*)

   B. *Simethicone*

   C. *Anticholinergics*

   D. None

   Answer: D

References

1. Roberts DM, Ostapchuk M, O'Brien JG. Infantile Colic. *American Family Physician* Volume 70 • Number 4 • August 15, 2004 735-740.
2. Weissbluth M. Colic. In: Burg FD, Gellis SS, Kagan BM. *Gellis & Kagan's Current pediatric therapy.* 16th ed. Philadelphia: Saunders, 1999:674–8
3. Garrison MM, Christakis DA. A systematic review of treatments for infant colic. *Pediatrics* 2000;106(1 pt 2):184–90

4. Lucassen PL, Assendelft WJ, Gubbels JW, van Eijk JT, van Geldrop WJ, Neven AK. Effectiveness of treatments for infantile colic: systematic review. [published erratum appears in BMJ 1998;317:171.] *BMJ* 1998;316:1563–9.
5. Metcalf TJ, Irons TG, Sher LD, Young PC. Simethicone in the treatment of infant colic: a randomized, placebo-controlled, multicenter trial. *Pediatrics* 1994;94:29–34.

Toxicologic Emergencies

Ryan Young, MD
Department of Pediatrics
The University of Arizona School of Medicine
Farshad, "Mazda" Shirazi, MS, MD, PhD, FACEP
Assistant Professor of Emergency Medicine
Toxicology & Pharmacology
The University of Arizona School of Medicine

Critical Knowledge

General Approach

Initial Life Support

- Remember ABCD's: airway patency, protective reflexes (gag reflex), adequate air entry, perfusion, GCS, think about an IV, ABG, FSBG, and oxygen initially
- Skin decontamination or eye flush for topical caustic agents
- GI decontamination: (possibly effective if within 10 minutes) the airway must be protected due to risk of aspiration or esophageal tear. Currently there is no evidence that the application of decontamination to remove toxins has any effect on the course. It is important to contact the poison control center nearest you if this is considered as an option in the management of an acute intoxication. Absolute contraindication in the ingestion of corrosive substances or hydrocarbons.
- Activated charcoal: the consensus understanding since 2004 is that activated charcoal does not alter the course of most toxicities. It is important to contact your poison control center if this is considered as an option for management. Contraindicated in: bowel obstruction or perforation, and aspiration, hypernatremia or hypermagnesemia.
- Whole bowel irrigation: osmotically balanced polyethylene glycol electrolyte solution 30 ml/kg/hr up to 500 ml/hr until stool is clear. Contraindicated in: caustic ingestion, hydrocarbon ingestion, foreign body, ileus or bowel perforation.

One Pill Kills

Drugs that may be fatal for a 10 kg child upon ingestion of one commercially available dose unit (at 1 year of age an infant can grasp a single pill with a pincer grasp, but only later has the ability to manage a handful of pills).

Drug	Symptoms	Management
Iron pills	Phases 1. (6 hours) mucosal injury- n/v, diarrhea, GI blood loss 2. (6-24hours) recovery-child appears well 3. (>24hours) metabolic acidosis, coma, seizures, shock	ABC's, labs: serum FE levels >500 ug risk for phase III UGI x-ray, whole bowel irrigation, IV *defuroxamine* 15 mg/kg/hr
Beta blockers, Ca+ Channel Blockers	Bradycardia, hypotension, AV block, hypoglycemia with BB's, and hyperglycemia with metabolic acidosis in CCB's	ABC's, *atropine*, fluid bolus, pressors, charcoal, *calcium* infusion for CCB"s
Clonidine	Altered mental status, lethargy, hypothermia, miosis, respiratory depression, coma	ABC's, resp. support, activated charcoal, *narcan*
Hypoglycemics (*Glucophage*)	Hypoglycemia, lethargy, metabolic acidosis	ABC's, charcoal, infusion of *hypertonic glucose, octreotide* 1-2 μg per kg per dose q6hrs
Theophyline	Headache, seizures, PVC's, tachycardia, extra systoles, arrhythmias	ABC's, close monitoring, antiarrhythmics, seizure precautions
Methylsalicylate (Icy Hot, oil of wintergreen – also a nontoxic *hydrocarbon*)	Cerebral edema, coma, lethargy, seizures, tinnitus, electrolyte imbalance, pulmonary edema	ABC's, close monitoring, correction of fluid and electrolyte imbalances, if severe hemodialysis or hemoperfusion.

Evaluation

- Six hour rule: "If nothing has occurred during the first 6 hours after ingestion, nothing will happen." The few exceptions to this rule include *acetaminophen*, hydrocarbon ingestion, and delayed release pharmaceuticals.
- History
    1. If known intoxication: (**4 E's**) **E**stimate amount, **E**lapsed time since ingestion, **E**arly symptoms, **E**arly interventions by patient or family
    2. If suspected but unknown intoxication: timing of onset, symptoms, medications at home, recent illness treatments, visitors, travel, acute altered mental status
       Note: if history is unknown admit and observe overnight.
- Physical exam: VS, GCS, skin-color, bullae, piloerection, diaphoresis, eyes-pupils, EOMI, fundi, mouth-odors, CV-perfusion, resp-air entry, rate, GI-motility
- Labs: consider: CBC, ABG, EKG, CXR, KUB, CMP-lytes, bun/cr, gluc, lft, urinalysis, rapid tox screen, and complete tox screen once a substance has been suspected through history
- All females of reproductive age should receive a pregnancy test
- All patients with a suspected toxicity should have *aspirin* and *acetaminophen* levels obtained
- Drugs that may need dialysis: (**AA STUMBLE**) **A**lcohol (Isopropyl) and **A**tenolol, **S**alicylates, **T**heophyline, **U**remia, **M**ethanol, **B**arbituates, **L**ithium/heavy metals, **E**thanol/**E**thylene glycol
- Radiopaque Toxins: (**CHIPES**) **C**hloral **H**ydrate, **H**eavy metals, **I**ron, **P**henothiazines, **E**nteric coating, **S**alycilates
- Seizure inducing toxicities: check Po2, and *glucose* and suspect *gyometra* (mushroom), heavy metals (arsenic, lead, mercury), sympathomimetics (*cocaine*, *amphetamines*), *B blockers*, TCA antidepressants, SSRI's, *methylhydrozine* or *isoniazide* treat with *pyradoxime*, SNAT, masses or consider fever especially if history is unknown

Critical Concepts and Management

Common Ingestions

- Acetaminophen: hepatotoxicity occurs with ingestions >200 mg/kg. Liver damage occurs 18-24 hours after ingestion. Symptoms develop within 14hr after the toxic ingestion is reached unless extended release. Symptoms include: malaise, anorexia, emesis, diaphoresis, hepatomegaly, hyperbilirubinemia, elevated liver function tests, elevated PTT, oliguria, encephalopathy, hypoglycemia, coagulopathy, renal failure.
    - Management: none needed if ingestion is less than 140-150 mg/kg and asymptomatic. Obtain *acetaminophen* level at least 4 hours after ingestion (best if obtained between 4-10 hours after ingestion). Compare the levels to the nomogram.
    - **Treat immediately without levels**: if >6-8 hours after ingestion, severe symptoms, staggered overdoses, or extended release formulations.
    - Obtain *aspirin* level, 4 hour Tylenol level, baseline electrolytes, creatinine, liver functions, coagulation studies, and a UA.
    - If activated charcoal is considered please call your poison control center.
    - *N-acetyl cysteine*: if initiated within 8 hours reduces hepatic damage. NAC: 140 mg/kg PO loading dose. Repeat if patient vomits within one hour. If patient cannot tolerate PO consider FDA approved *acetadote* (NAC IV formulation): 150 mg/kg diluted in 200 ml 5% *dextrose* administered over 30-60 minutes to avoid anaphalactoid reaction. Then a maintenance dose of 50 mg/kg diluted in 500 ml 5% *dextrose* administered over 4 hours, followed by 100 mg/kg diluted in 1,000 ml 5 % *dextrose* over 16 hours. Theoretically *acetadote* administration may be less effective than PO. **Warning:** always call your poison control center to review the potential administration dose of NAC.
- Alcohols: *ethanol* is the most common. Symptoms include: nausea, vomiting, stupor, ataxia, coma, and death. Lethal concentrations are >500 mg/dl. Once levels exceed 50-100 mg/dl. Triad of: coma, hypothermia, and hypoglycemia, often accompanied by metabolic acidosis in children.
    - Management: *methanol* or *ethylene glycol*: *ethanol*-indicated if level is >20 mg/dl, competitively binds substrates. If HPI is concerning for

ingestion of *methanol* or *ethylene glycol* hydrate at 1.5 X maitenence fluids or give the first dose of *fomepizole* 15 mg/kg IV infusion over 30 min, then 10 mg/kg every 12 hours for x4 doses then 15 mg/kg q 12 hr until level is less than 20 mg/dl. If unsure about ingestion the first dose of *flomipizole* will buy you 12 hours to help aid your history.

- ▸ *Ethanol*: if seizures or *glucose* <60 then administer 10-12.5% IV *dextrose* (a 4 fold dilution of 50% *dextrose* will yield 12.5%) and use 2 ml/kg in children <50 kg. Hemodialysis if concentration >500 mg/dl.

- Anticholinergics: including antidepressants, antihistamines, antispasmodics, and belladonna alkaloids. Competitive antagonists with acetycholine at the neruoreceptor site. Symptoms remember: mad as a hatter (delirium), red as a beet (flushing), dry as a bone (dry mucous membranes), blind as a bat (mydriasis), and hot as a hare (hyperpyrexia).
    - ▸ Management: a universal effect of all drugs in this class is decreased GI motility so toxicity may be delayed up to 24 hours. Seizures: 0.1-0.2 mg/kg IV *diazepam.* Severe agitation with a clear anticholinergic toxidrome. A diagnostic dose of *physostigmine* 0.5 mg via IV infusion over 5 minutes with a repeat every 10 min for a max of 4 mg may be helpful. **Warning**: If to rapid or to large a dose (>4 mg), may precipitate seizures, or asystole. Watch for muscarinic toxicity (bronchospasm, bradycardia, hypertension, seizures) and antidote that with IV *atropine.* Always call your poison control center and consult a toxicologist before giving antidote or administration of *physostigmine.*
- Antidepressants: including TCA's, SSRI's and the rare MAOI's.
    - ▸ TCA's: are considered the most dangerous and precipitate seizures, arrhythmias (V-tach, V-fib), hypotension. Ingestion of >35 mg/kg may be fatal.
        - ▪ Management: ABC's, 12 lead EKG, cardiac monitor, NaHCO3 1-2 mEq/kg bolus maintain serum pH 7.45-7.55. Treat all arrhythmias with extra boluses of NaHCO3 (if EKG shows QRS >100 msec or R in AVR give x 1 bolus of 1-2 meq/kg of NaHCO3 and check to see if QRS narrows start a NaHCO3 drip with consultation with poison control, if the QRS does not narrow give another bolus). Always call poison control and obtain a toxicology consult.
    - ▸ SSRI's: beware serotonin syndrome: (co ingestion MAOI or *amphetamines*) seizures, muscle rigidity lower extremity >upper extremity, hyperpyrexia, clonus, tachycardia, cardiac arrhythmias, rhabdomyolysis, and flushing.

        - Management: supportive care, core temperature monitoring with foley temp if available, external cooling, sedatives, and airway management for hyperthermia up to 72 hours, *cyproheptadine* 0.25 mg/kg/24 hrs Q8 hours with max dose children 2-6 12 mg/24 hrs, and children 7-14 16 mg/24 hrs. Always call poison control and obtain a toxicology consult if serotonin syndrome is suspected.
    - MAOI's: ingestions of 6 mg/kg or more can be fatal. Also interact with tyramine (cheese, soy sauce, decongestants) causing seizure, stoke, or hypertension.
        - Management: 24 hours obs. Watch for rhabdo, hyperprexia, and hypertension. Treat muscle rigidity with benzos and neuromuscular blockade. Always call poison control and obtain a toxicology consult other therapies may be available including interlipid therapy.
- <u>*Aspirin*</u>: symptoms are wide ranging. Cerebral edema, coma, lethargy, seizures, tinnitus, and electrolyte imbalance. ABG: metabolic acidosis, with respiratory alkalosis however respiratory acidosis quickly develops because kids can not sustain such a high respiratory rate.
    - 150-300 mg/kg mild symptoms (GI upset, tachypnea, tinnitus)
    - 300-500 mg/kg moderate toxicity (agitation, fever, diaphoresis)
    - >500 mg/kg severe toxicity (seizure coma, dysarthia, pulm edema)
    - Management: ABC'S, cardiac monitoring, fluid therapy to restore hydration to prevent renal failure. Resuscitate with 2-3 normal *saline* bolus at 20 ml/kg. If *aspirin* level is >30 then initiate fluid alkalinization with 5% *dextrose* with 100-150 mEq per L of NaHCO3 with 20 meq/kg *potassium* at 1-1.5 X maitenence for a total of eight hours. The goal is to produce 10-2 ml/kg/hr of urine output and urine ph >7.5. Repeat *salycilate* level in 4-6 hours after initiation and always consult your poison control center for recommendations on fluid management. Hemodialysis is indicated if unresponsive acidosis, lyte disturbances, seizures, coma, or plasma *salicylate* level >100 mg/dl for acute ingestions, or >60 mg/dl for chronic.
- <u>*Barbituates*</u> and <u>*Benzodiazepines*</u>: (CNS sedative, hypnotics) measure *phenobarb* levels 1-2 hours after ingestion. Remember *pentobarbital* does not show up on *Phenobarbital* toxicity tests you must request the lab to look for this. Pt. has sluggishness, dysarhria, poor memory, emotional lability, irritability, and emotional lability. Also very dependant drugs with withdrawal showing tremulousness, agitation, or convulsions.

- Management: ABC's and supportive care are the standard. Always consult poison control before giving *flumazenil* for *benzodiazepine* overdose: 0.01-0.02 mg/kg IV (max 0.2 mg/dose) can repeat to max 0.05 mg/kg (total max 1 mg) as antidote may force patient into withdrawal.

- *Beta Blockers*: overdose is most common with *atenolol*. Symptoms include seizure, altered mental status, cardiac arrhythmia (AV node blockade, accelerated junctional rhythms), decreased contractility, bradycardia, hypotension, respiratory depression, and bronchospasm (exacerbating previous asthma related conditions.
  - Management: cardiac monitor conduction delays and arrhythmias, IV Boluses 20 ml/kg, *glucagon* (for its inotrophic and vasopressor effects) 0.05-0.15 mg/kg IV bolus (max 10 mg) 0.05-0.1 mg/kg/hr infusion always administer with D5W fluid, utilize pressors as needed. Other therapies including interlipid may be available and indicated please call your poison control center.
- Botulism Toxin: usually from improperly home-canned low acidity vegetables, poorly refrigerated meats, and recorded incidence of karo syrup. Incubation is 12-36 hours with symptoms ranging from malaise, diplopia, dysphagia (gag reflex), and dysarthria. PE reveals, lateral rectus weakness, ptosis, and papillary abnormalities. Diagnosis is clinical.
  - Management: serum and stool analysis, suggestive EMG findings. Supportive care of airway and ventilation status. Trivalent antitoxin is used and available form the CDC it is important to consult a toxicologist and inform your poison control center to facilitate the use of Baby BIG.
- *Ca Channel Blockers*: overdose most common with *verapamil*. Symptoms may develop hours after ingestion and the most morbidity occurs with sustained release formulations, *verapamil*, or *diltiazem*. Symptoms include seizure, altered mental status, cardiac arrhythmia (AV node blockade, accelerated junctional rhythms), decreased contractility, bradycardia, hypotension, peripheral vasodilatation, apnea, pulmonary edema, bowel infarction, lactic acidosis, hyperglycemia, mild hyperkalemia, flushing, and peripheral cyanosis. *Nifedipine* is known to give seizures.
  - Management: ABC's, IV hydration starting with NS bolus 20ml/kg, don't induce emesis as the vagal stimulus may induce a heart block. Cardiac monitoring, *glucagon* (for its inotrophic and vasopressor effects) 0.05-0.15mg/kg IV bolus (max 10mg) 0.05-0.1mg/kg/hr infusion always administer with D5W fluid. *Atropine* for hypotension

and if unresponsive administer *calcium* salts 10 ml of 10% CaCl (if pt has a central line or in a code situation) or 30 ml of 10% *calcium gluconoate* (preferred if pt is not coding) which may be repeated x 2-3 as necessary. If all therapies fail there is evidence that simultaneous administration of *insulin* and *glucose* can help provided that *serum glucose* is maintained around 100mg/dl. If this is considered or pressors are needed please call poison control of a check of doses and additional instructions.

- Carbamazepine: a very common pediatric overdose. Symptoms include: motor restlessness, tremor, athetosis, mydriasis, nystagmus, cardiac conduction abnormalities, respiratory depression, and twitching.
  - Management: ABC's, due to the delayed gastric emptying effect of the drug multiple doses of charcoal are indicated. *Carbamazepine* level is useful if obtained 2-4 hours after ingestion but may not indicate level of toxicity. This is an exception to the previous activated charcoal instruction. Activated charcoal is indicated to eliminate cyclic absorption and coma at 1 g/kg po or per NG tube q 1-6 hours up to 100 gms. Always watch for aspiration and contact your poison control center for instructions.
- Carbon Monoxide: accounts for the largest group of poisoning deaths among children. A product of incomplete combustion, it has 210x more affinity for *oxygen*. Thus a left shift of the *oxygen* dissociation curve which results in decreased *oxygen* delivery to tissues. It is an odorless, colorless, and tasteless gas. Pts with 20% of hb affected complain of headache and nausea. Pts. with 20-40% tire and become confused, and involvement in >40% result in ataxia, collapse, arrhythmias, cerebral edema, acidosis, and coma. **Note**: consider CO poisoning in any patient during winter with a headache and/or nausea.
  - Management: ABC's, conscious patient give 100% oxygen using nonrebreather face mask at 10 lpm until COHb is <10% and symptoms resolve. Remember SaO2 is not accurate. Measure carboxyhemoglobin levels in the blood. Elimination half life is 4-6 hours on RA and 1 hour with 100% oxygen. ECG and CXR are helpful to evaluate for heart attack, pneumonitis, atalectasis, or pulm edema. *Hyperbaric oxygen* should be considered if evidence of cardiac abnormalities and high COHb concentrations, seizure, coma, pregnancy. Always call your poison control center, and obtain a toxicologist referral immediately this will facilitate a speedy transition to such therapy.

- *Clonidine*: stimulates CNS a2-adrenergic receptors. Typical dose of 100-200 ug in adults therefore as above small amounts can be lethal. Symptoms include altered mental status from lethargy to coma, hypothermia, miosis, and respiratory depression. Intoxication typically lasts 8-24 hours.
  - Management: ABC's, charcoal, hemodynamic management, *Naloxone* 1-2 mg as a trial may be effective. Always call your poison control center before administration and obtain a toxicology consult. Chronic use with administration of antidote can cause a possible fatal emergency.
- *Digoxin*: has a very appealing color to the elixir. Inhibits the Na-K ATPase. Two toxicities: acute (usually a toddler ingesting a relative's medication) and chronic (usually a toddler that has a congenital heart disease). Chronic ingestions are more likely to be toxic. Acute ingestions may have no clinically observable effects. The most common and earliest symptom may be nausea, commonly followed by bradycardia. Complete absorption is achieved in 2-4 hours. Other symptoms include: lethargy, headache, disorientation, visual disturbances (haloes of color), heart block and AV node disassociation, ventricular or supraventricular escape rhythms, emesis, anorexia, and hyperkalemia.
  - Management: ABC's, levels are most useful if measured 4-6 hours post ingestion. Serum digoxin toxicity is generally 4 mg/ml however toxicity is clinical based on pharmacokinetics. Cardiac monitoring is important, and electrolyte disturbances are important to monitor and treat. Most toxicity symptoms are based on electrolyte imbalance. *Digoxin*-specific antibody fragments are indicated for progressing clinical toxicity, arrhythmias with end organ damage, or serum K >5.5 mEq/l. The dose is calculated in vials by
    - # vials = known ingested dose/0.6

      OR if known ingested dose is not known
    - # vials = SDC (ng/ml) X wt (kg)/100
  - Always consult your poison control center to check these calculations and for any patient who has any history of heart disease or previous use of *digoxin*.
  - Complications include: allergic reaction, precipitation of congestive heart failure due to the loss of inotropic support of *digoxin*, and rebound hypokalemia. Give infusions over 30 minutes via a 0.22 μm inline filter.

- Disc batteries: usually children 4-8 yrs old. Often contain mercury, lithium, and KOH, and have a corrosive effect on the mucosal surfaces they contact.
  - Management: ABC's, CXR, if the battery is in the esophagus then they must be removed, if not then the object is likely expelled within 72 hours and no intervention is necessary. The pyloris has a limit of <9 mm for passage of the battery.
- Hydrocarbons: known also as petroleum distillates, spread over large surface areas such as the lungs. Symptoms include coughing, gagging, choking, drooling, tachypnea, altered mental status, or vomiting. Toxic hydrocarbons include: halogenated (*carbon tetrachloride, trichloroethane*), aromatic (*benzene, toluene, xylene*), additive (*camphor, organophospates*, heavy metals), turpentine, basoline, kerosene, lighter fluid, and mineral spirits.
  - Management: ABC's, respiratory support, skin and eye decontamination is extremely important consult poison control of appropriate methods. If symptomatic obtain CXR and admit for 12-24 hour obs. If CXR normal then repeat in 2-4 hours if normal can discharge in 4 hours if asymptomatic. If there is any question of delayed pneumonitis it is best to admit the patient to an inpatient facility and obtain a toxicology consult.
- Lead: major source is lead based paint used in 1950's. The most common modern presentation is declining mental status, or acute onset of poor performance in school. Symptoms of plumbism include: abdominal complaints, colicky pain, constipation, anorexia, vomiting, listlessness, sudden onset disability, or cognitive deficit. Encaphalopathy is shown by persistent vomiting, fatigue, clumsiness, or ataxia with declining mental status. A sensitive measure of the effect of lead on heme synthesis is **E**rythrocyte **P**rotoporphyrin (**EP**) a heme precursor that can be measured in the blood. Levels 250-300 ug in the blood is very likely chronic lead poisoning. X-ray of extremities may show lead deposition.
  - Management: lead level 20-44 ug/dl confirmed by an EP of >250 ug/dl. Environmental investigation, toxicologist referral, and chelation therapy. Seizures should be controlled with standard anticonvulsant drugs. Aggressive management of ICP. It is a good idea to consult poison control for guidance if contemplating chelation therapy.

Guidelines for Chelation Therapy		
Encephalopathy	BAL 450 $mg/m^2/d$ + $CaNa_2EDTA$ 1,500 $mg/m^2/d$	75 mg/m^2 IM every 4 hr for 5 days Continuous infusion or 2-4 divided IV doses for 5 days (start 4 hours after BAL)
Symptomatic with Blood Lead >70	BAL 300-450 $mg/m^2/d$ + $CaNa_2EDTA$ 1,000-1,500 $mg/m^2/d$	50-75 mg/m^2 IM every 4 hr for 3-5 days Continuous infusion or 2-4 divided IV doses for 5 days (start 4 hours after BAL)
Asymptomatic with Blood Lead 45-69	Succimer 700-1,050 $mg/m^2/d$ Or $CaNa_2EDTA$ 1,000 $mg/m^2/d$	8-10 mg/kg TID for 5 days, then BID for 14 days Continuous infusion or 2-4 divided IV doses for 5 days

- Organophosphates (cholinergics): insecticides found in agriculture and home use. Usually inhaled, ingested, or with skin penetration. Symptoms are present during the first 12 hours after contact and involve the CNS. They include: dizziness, headache, ataxia, and convulsions. (**DUMBELS**) **D**iarrhea, **U**rination, **M**iosis, **B**ronchospasm, **B**radycardia, **B**ronchorrhea, **E**mesis, **L**acrimation, **S**alivation.
    - Management: if oral use gastric lavage taking care to avoid exposure to expelled fluid. Scrub thoroughly with soap on skin and mucous membranes, and immediately remove contaminated clothing. *Atropine sulfate* 0.05-0.1 mg/kg and 2-5 mg for teens and adults. Repeat every 10-30 min prn until all absorbed chemical has been metabolized (warning may require up to 2,000 mg of *atropine* over several days). *Pralicoxime* 25-50 mg/kg in 250 ml *saline* over 30 min should be used for symptoms of profound weakness, and muscle twitching. Can repeat doses at 1 hour intervals if the symptoms are not relieved. Remember end point is relief if symptoms. Also hydrocarbon solutions are used with organophosphates to treat in order to avoid bronchopulmonary pneumonia.

- Plants: Very common ingestions

Plant	Symptoms	Management
Laburnum	Vomiting, pallor, dilated pupils, tachycardia, dizziness	ABC's, observation and supportive care
Atropa Belladona (deadly nightshade)	Dry mouth, dilated pupils, hallucinations, urinary retention, agitation, ataxia, convulsions	ABC's, observation and supportive care
Laurel	GI upset, salivation, flushing, convulsions, arrhythmias. Symptoms can be delayed 4 hours.	Unless broken seeds or chewing no intervention. ABC's, observation and supportive care for broken seeds.
Lupin		Nontoxic unless large quantities, ABC's, observation and supportive care
Yew Tree	Nausea, vomiting, anticholinergic effects, drowsiness, bradycardia, arrhythmias, convulsions	Obs for 4 hours (asymptomatic), supportive treatments
Woody Nightshade	Drowsiness, ataxia, nausea, vomiting oropharyngeal irritation	If >5 berries or any unripe berries ABC's, observation and supportive care. Obs for 8 hours (asymptomatic)
Cuckoo pint	Mucosal irritation, edema, skin irritation and blistering	Analgesia and antihistamines for symptoms
Elder	Nausea, vomiting, dizziness, tachycardia, confusions	Symptomatic only, ABC's, observation and supportive care
Mistletoe	Nausea, vomiting, diarrhea, muscle weakness, pupil dilation, diuresis, bradycardia	>3 berries for symptoms, ABC's, observation and supportive care, *atropine* for bradycardia
Rhubarb	Gastric irritation, hypocalcemia	Milk, and ABC's, observation and supportive care

- Mushrooms: two types of species
  - Immediate onset: symptoms within 6 hours of ingestion. Usually cause muscarinic effects: sweat, salivation, colic, and pulmonary edema. Use *atropine*. Other early onset mushrooms cause anticholinergic effects with mania and hallucinations use supportive care and monitoring of fluid status.
  - Delayed onset: >6 hours: 90% of all related deaths. Symptoms Include: GI upset, fever, tachycardia, hyperglycemia, and 24 hours after ingestion fulminant hepatic failure. Without liver transplant patients will di.e., GI decontamination, and activated charcoal, consult mycologist if available.
- Drugs of Abuse

Drug	Symptoms	Management
Amphetamines (includes caffeine, *pseudo-ephedrine*, energy drinks etc)	Dilated and reactive pupils, hyperthermia, confusion, hallucinations, irritability, delusions, hyperacute sensorium, paranoid ideation, euphoria, pressured speech, hyperactivity, hypertensive crisis, anorexia, rhabdomyolysis, bladder sphincter contraction, flushing, dry mouth	Activated charcoal, *benzos* or *haldol* for agitation and seizures. Treat hypertension with *hydralazine*, or *sodium nutroprusside* IV. Maintain urine output. Treat rhabdomyolysis with IV fluids and urinary alkalinization. External cooling measures for hyperthermia. Detectable in blood or urine 48 after use.
Cocaine	Insomnia, seizure, stoke, pressured speech, muscle rigidity, dilated pupils, agitation, euphoria, paranoid delusions, hallucinations, aggression, tachycardia, tachyarrhythmias, heart attack, renal failure, rhabdomyolisis, diaphoresis, flushing. **Infants**: dystonic posturing, seizures, hyperactivity, altered mental status **Withdrawal**: depression, cravings, with symptoms peak-ing 2-3 days after last use	Seizures, tachycardia, and hypertensive crisis treat with benzos. Also use nitroprusside to prevent heart attack and stoke. Serial ECG's, and hyperthermia with external cooling. Head CT for stoke. Diuresis if rhabdomyolysis or myoglobinuria. Detected in urine up to 3 days after last use.

Drug	Symptoms	Management
Ecstasy	Three Stages 1. Disorientation 2. Tingling, spasmodic jerking 3. Distortion, illusions, overly sociable. Stoke, tremor, tics, ataxia, nystagmus, insomnia, malignant hyperthermia, mydriasis, confusion, agitation, liver failure, jaw clenching, dehydration, DIC, rhabdomyolysis **Withdrawal**: fatigue, myalgias, poor concentration, confusion, anxiety, insomnia	External cooling for hyperthermia. Hypertension treated with sedation nitroprusside, and *Ca-channel-blockers*. Activated charcoal. Usually not detectable in urine screens use gas chromatography and mass spec. Present in urine up to 16 hours after ingestion.
Gamma Hydoxybutyrate (GHB), date rape drug, also used for anabolic uses to increase muscle mass	Sudden onset coma is the most common presentation Onset in 15 minutes with peak in 20-60 min effects last 6-8 hrs and prolonged with ETOH. Seizure, CNS depression, sedation, tremor, nystagmus, miosis, ataxia, hypothermia, aggression, bradycardia, hypo tension **Withdrawal**: feeling of doom	Supportive, *atropine* for bradycardia, GI lavage and charcoal not indicated due to the rapidity of absorption. Undetectable in urine, mass spec and gas chromatography indicated.
Hallucinogens: *mescaline, magic mushrooms, LSD, PCP* Half life=1-3 days	Psychosis, disinhibition, euphoria, anxiety, paranoia, mood lability, thought distortions, hyperreflexia, dilated pupils, tachycardia, flushing. LSD: flashbacks, psychosis with hyperalertness, delusions of grandeur, visual perception distortion, parathesias, weakness. PCP: seizures, cyclic coma, ataxia, blank stare, muscle rigidity, dystonia, tardive dyskinesia, aggression, analgesia, violence, amnesia.	*Benzodiazepines* for seizures, *Haldol* for anxiety and chemical restraint (physical restraints should be avoided), decrease stimulation for the patient. Check uric acid, CPK, *creatinine*, liver enzymes for rhabdomyolysis. Enzyme-multiple immunoassay technique for pcp test.

Drug	Symptoms	Management
Ketamine	Nystagmus, analgesia, anxiety, sedation, amnesia, disordered thought, hallucination, tachycardia, hypertension, rhabdomyolisis	Treat agitation with *benzos*. Monitor lytes and *creatinine* maintain hydration for rhabdomyolysis. About 2 hours after presentation if patient returns to baseline can d/c home. Not detected by routine tox screens. Use high-performance liquid chromatography.
Marijuana: smoking is x3 more potent than enteral	Ataxia, dysarthria, euphoria, anxiety, time-space distortion, delusions, confusion, respiratory distress with airway obstruction, dry mucous membranes. Peak 2-3 hours after ingestion.	For delirium or anxiety use *benzos*. Can detect in urine up to 3 days after use. *Trazodone* for disabling insomnia (withdrawal)
Opioids	Seizures, coma, stupor, analgesia, emotional lability, anxiolysis, sedation, pinpoint pupils, cyanosis, hypothermia, hyporeflexia, decreased gastric HCL and pancreatic secretions, constipation, increased anal sphincter tone, miosis IV: septic emboli, endocarditis, abcesses **Withdrawal**: insomnia, agitation, irritability, piloerection	*Naloxone* 0.2-0.4 and titrate upward slowly, *Methadone* to prevent withdrawal. Can be detected up to 3 days post ingestion.

Note: this chapter is designed as a guide for treatment, and an aid for acute toxicologic emergencies. It is not the definitive or complete source of information. Your local poison control center should be consulted with any questions and often to simply double check management.

Questions

1. A five year old male is brought to the ED after a suspected overdose. While in a private care on the way over, the patient has "shaking movements" and is seen to have tonic clonic activity while presenting to triage. Which of the following is less likely to be associated with seizures?

   A. *Opioids*

   B. *B blockers*

   C. *Anticholinergics*

   D. *Sympathomimetics*

   E. Acute heavy metal ingestion

   Answer: A. *Opioids* are less likely to cause seizures in pediatric patients. The other choices are associated with seizure in acute intoxication.

2. A 4 year old male with a known seizure disorder presents to the ED with acute mental status change. Father states the patient has been irritable for a couple of weeks. During the morning he was unable to wake from sleep, and was unresponsive to voice and stimulation. Upon arrival in the ED the patient is obtunded, having agonal breathing, with a GCS of 8, moaning only to painful stimulus. After the initial ABC's the patient is intubated and put on a CV monitor, IV access is obtained, and the patient is resuscitated. The patient has a temp of 36.4, a BMP shows *sodium* of 118 and the patient has a very brisk urine output. You suspect SIADH. What toxidrome can give you the above symptoms?

   A. *Benzodiazepines*

   B. *ACE inhibitors*

   C. *Anticholinergics*

   D. *Tegretol*

   E. *Phenobarbital*

   Answer: D. *Carbamazepime* is associated with these symptoms. Also the fact the child has a known seizure disorder helps to sort out the symptoms.

3. A nine year old boy is brought to the ED after he was found in his family's farm confused and disoriented. He presents having urinated his pants, doubled over holding his stomach, and with multiple bouts of emesis. Upon physical exam he is wheezing with respiratory distress, has moist skin, muscle twitching, and miosis bilaterally. What is the best management for this patient after ABCD's?

   A. ABC's, remove clothing, *atropine* and *pralixocime* until symptoms resolve

B. ABC's, activated charcoal, *benzos* or *haldol*, IV fluids with alkalinization, and cooling measures
C. ABC's, gastric lavage, UGI x-ray, whole bowel irrigation, IV *defuroxamine* 15 mg/kg/hr
D. ABC's, serial EKG's, *glucagon*, and respiratory support
E. ABC's, supportive care, *diazepam* for seizures, external cooling, sedatives, and airway management for hyperthermia up to 72 hours

Answer: A. This is the classic pesticide exposure. Skin decontamination is key along with *atropine* as an antidote. Gastric lavage and charcoal are rarely indicated

4. A 12 month old girl is hospitalized for ingesting what mom thinks is approximately two tablespoons of vitamin E oil. You observe her for approximately 6 hours and perform a chest x-ray which is normal. At this point the best decision is to

   A. Gastric lavage, with whole bowel irrigation
   B. Send her home with close follow up
   C. Hospitalize and observe overnight with serial chest Xrays
   D. Trial her on room air for another three hours if no symptoms then send her home
   E. Supportive care, with PICU admission for possible pneumonitis

   Answer: C. The HPI is not firm on what is going on. The six hour rule often does not apply to hydrocarbon ingestions as they can cause a delayed pneumonitis. It is best to observe in an inpatient setting.

5. A 15 month old boy arrives in the ED lethargic, with poor respiratory effort, and a slight tremor. The boys' parents are divorced and the father administered a medication for the first time that evening. He knows that his son was recently hospitalized for an extended period of time and was intubated for acute respiratory failure. What is the next step in management of this child?

   A. Intubate, provide supportive care, and admit to the PICU
   B. Administer the appropriate dose of *flumazanil*
   C. Call poison control to consult
   D. Supportive care, *diazepam* for seizures, external cooling, sedatives, and airway management for hyperthermia up to 72 hours

E. Gastric lavage, UGI x-ray, whole bowel irrigation, IV *defuroxamine* 15 mg/kg/hr

Answer: C. Your local poison control center can help especially if the patient has a possible history of taking the drug in the past. Withdrawal is a real danger.

References

1. American Academy of Pediatrics Committee on Drugs: *Acetaminophen* toxicity in children. *Pediatrics* 2001;108 (4): 1020-1024.
2. Ford MD, Delaney KA, Ling LL, Erickson T (eds): *Clinical Toxicology*, 1st ed. Philadelphia, WB Sounders, 2001
3. Jones AL: J *Toxicology* 1998;36:277-285. Tylenol nomogram.
4. Miller K, Chang A: Acute inhalation injury. *Emerg Med Clin North Am* 2003;21 (2):533-557.
5. Ousterhoudt KC, Shannon M, Henretig FM: *Toxicologic emergencies.* In Fleisher GR, Ludwig S (eds): Textbook of Pediatric Emergency Medicine, 4th ed. Philadelphia, Lippincott Williams & Wilkins, 2006.
6. Riordan M, Rylance G, Berry K. *Poisoning in children 1: General Management.* Arch Dis Child 2002;87:392-396.
7. Riordan M, Rylance G, Berry K. *Poisoning in children 4: Household products, plants, and mushrooms.* Arch Dis Child 2002;87:403-406.
8. Riordan M, Rylance G, Berry K. *Poisoning in children 5 rare and dangerous poisons.* Arch Dis Child 2002;87:407-410.
9. Tenenbein, M. Poisoning pearls regarding the very young. *Clin Ped Emerg Med* 2000;1:176-179.
10. Temple AR: *Acute and chronic effects of aspirin toxicity and their treatment.* Arch Intern Med 1981;141:366.

Urinary Tract Infections

Abby L. Jones, MD
Emergency Medicine/Pediatrics Combined Resident
Department of Emergency Medicine and Pediatrics
University of Maryland

Critical Knowledge

- **U**rinary **T**ract **I**nfection (**UTI**) is the single most common serious bacterial infection in infants.
- Accounts for approximately 5% of fever in children under 1 year of age.[1]
- Underdiagnosis of urinary tract infection in infants may lead to renal scarring, hypertension, and renal insufficiency as infections in this age group may be the result of anatomical abnormalities.[2]
- Urinary tract infections are treated differently based on the age of the child.[2]

Background/Epidemiology/Anatomy

- Urinary tract infections account for approximately 5% of febrile episodes in infants less than 1 year old.[1]
- Boys are more likely to have urinary tract infections during the first 3 months of life; then the prevalence shifts to females for the remainder of their lives.
- The body's natural defense against urinary tract infections is to empty the bladder regularly and completely. Any abnormality in the urinary tract which limits or inhibits this function leads to a greater likelihood of urinary tract infections.
- Vesicoureteral reflux may be present in up to 30-50% of children diagnosed with urinary tract infections.[3]

Diagnosis/Differential

- Fever may be the only presenting symptom in infants with urinary tract infections.
- Young infants presenting with a fever (temperature greater than 38°C or 100.4°F) should be evaluated for the presence of a serious bacterial infection including meningitis, bacteremia, cellulitis, osteomyelitis, and urinary tract infection.

- Certain subgroups of older infants (greater than 3 months) and toddlers should be evaluated for urinary tract infections even in the absence of urinary symptoms (as urinary symptoms may be difficult or impossible to illicit in this age group). These include highly febrile (temperature greater than 102.2°F) girls less than 1 year old, highly febrile (temp >102.2°F) circumcised boys less than 6 mo old, and highly febrile (temp >102.2) uncircumcised boys less than 1 year old.[4]
- In older children with complaints of abdominal pain and dysuria, the differential of renal calculi, vulvovaginitis, and urethritis from STDs should be considered. If fever is also present, appendicitis should be added to the list.

Critical Concepts

- Culture is the "gold-standard" to diagnosis. Diagnosis of a urinary tract infection should be made through urinalysis and urine culture where the former can be negative at the time of evaluation.
- "Bagged" urine is not appropriate for infants who are not yet potty-trained, their urines should be obtained by catheterization.
- A suprapubic aspiration should not be obtained routinely because of the degree of invasiveness, and should only be used in situations where catheterized urine is not possible (i.e., hypospadia, adhesions).
- Urine may be obtained from a potty-trained infant/toddler via clean catch, and the parents should be instructed on the proper method of cleaning prior to retrieval.
- A screening macroscopic urinalysis should be evaluated for the presence of nitrites and leukocyte esterase (an indirect test for bacteria and leukocytes, respectively).
- Microscopic analysis should routinely be performed in infants irrespective of the macroscopic analysis. Microscopic analysis allows the identification of leukocytes, bacteria, and epithelial cells (an indication of contamination) that may be present.
- Urine culture should be considered positive for >100,000 colony forming units on a clean catch specimen or >10,000 colony forming units from a catheterized specimen.

Treatment

- Treatment of urinary tract infections is dependent on the age of the child.
- Infants less than two month of age with a urinary tract infection should be admitted and treated with IV antibiotics (*ampicillin* and *cefotaxime* or *ampicillin* and *gentamicin*) initially. They may be transitioned to an outpatient oral course of antibiotics at the discretion of the admitting MD. This is usually after a sepsis rule out is complete and the patient has remained afebrile. Oral therapy should be tailored to the culture and sensitivity of the urine. The total duration of therapy should be two weeks.
- Infants between one and three months of age who appear acutely ill should be admitted and treated similarly to infants less than one month of age (their antibiotic therapy should include a third generation *cephalosporin* and *gentamicin*).
- With E. coli being a significant cause of CNS infection in neonates, consider a lumbar puncture in all children under one month of age and ill children under two months of age.
- Infants between one and three months of age who are not acutely ill may be managed as outpatients under the discretion of the emergency physician. Their course of therapy should be 10 to 14 days.
- Older children with cystitis may be managed on oral antibiotics as outpatients. Therapy should be tailored to the sensitivities determined by the urine.
- Empiric treatment may be started prior to the culture results based on the regional bacterial sensitivities. Commonly used antibiotics include: *amoxicillin* and *trimethoprin/sulfamethoxazole*. A test of cure should be considered if there is indication of treatment failure. Treatment of a UTI in a child should be for 10 days.
- Pyelonephritis may be treated either as an inpatient or outpatient, depending on certain patient related factors. In order to be a candidate for outpatient management, the child must be non-toxic appearing, able to tolerate oral medications without vomiting, be free of severe obstructing or refluxing uropathy, and compliant with treatment. These patients may be treated with a 10-14 day course of an oral third generation *cephalosporin*. Children with persistent fever after the third day of treatment or those who can no longer tolerate oral therapy (i.e., pt begins vomiting) should be reassessed for inpatient admission.

Follow-up Imaging

- Follow up imaging is indicated for all first time urinary tract infections in boys regardless of age and in girls less than 5 years old. Recurrent urinary tract infections in girls greater than 5 years old also necessitate further imaging.
- A renal ultrasound should be performed to evaluate for abnormalities of the urinary tract (i.e., cystic/dysplastic kidneys, duplicating collecting systems, renal scarring).
- A **V**oiding **C**ysto**U**rethro**G**ram (**VCUG**) should be performed once the acute episode is over and the urine has been cleared of bacteria. This test determines the presence of vesicoureteral reflux and the severity of the reflux if present (grade 1-5).
- It is the responsibility of the ED physician to inform the parents of the importance and need for follow up imaging when a urinary tract infection is diagnosed in the emergency department.

References

1. Hoberman A, Chao HP, Keller DM, et al. Prevalence of urinary tract infection in febrile infants. *J Pediatr* 1993; 123, 17.
1. American Academy of Pediatrics. Practice parameter: the diagnosis, treatment, and evaluation of the initial urinary tract infection in febrile infants and young children. American Academy of Pediatrics. Committee on Quality Improvement. Subcommittee on Urinary Tract Infection. *Pediatrics* 1999;103:843-52
2. Weiss R, Tamminen-Mobius T, Koskimies O, et al. Characteristics at entry of children with severe primary vesicoureteral reflux recruited for a multicenter, international therapeutic trial comparing medical and surgical management. The International Reflux Study in Children. *J Urol*; 1992, 148, 1644.
3. Baraff L. Management of fever without a source in infants and children. *Ann Em Med.* 2000: 36: 602-614.

Urological Emergencies

Edwin F. Lopez, MD
Department of Emergency Medicine
Wayne State University/Sinai-Grace Hospital
Detroit, MI

The Acute Hemiscrotum

The three leading differentials to consider in the atraumatic acute hemiscrotum include testicular torsion, epididymitis, and torsion of the appendix testis or appendix epididymis.

Testicular Torsion

Critical Knowledge

- A true urologic emergency
- Twisting and strangulation of the spermatic cord results in loss of blood supply to the testicle, leading to ischemia and necrosis
- The typical history is an acute, unilateral, painful and swollen hemiscrotum. It often presents during the nighttime. Beware, as complaints may also include vague abdominal discomfort or intermittent pain lasting from hours to days.
- Systemic symptoms are common, especially nausea and vomiting
- Remember, "castration by procrastination." If this diagnosis is considered, immediate urology consultation is mandatory from the emergency department.
- Always consider doing a genital exam in patients complaining of abdominal pain regardless of age

Epidemiology/Anatomy

- Incidence is bimodal with peaks during infancy and between 12-18 years of age
- An abnormal attachment of the tunica vaginalis results in a predisposition for testicular torsion
- Physical exam may reveal a high riding testicle with a transverse lie as opposed to the normal vertical lie
- The entire testicle will be exquisitely tender and swollen making it difficult to distinguish from orchitis and epididymo-orchitis

Differential Diagnosis

- Torsion of the Appendix Testis and Appendix Epididymis
- Epididymitis
- Orchitis
- Hydrocele, Varicocele
- Hernia
- Trauma
- Tumor

Diagnosis

- This is primarily a clinical diagnosis based on history and physical findings suggestive of torsion
- Lack of the ipsilateral cremasteric reflex is sensitive but not specific for the diagnosis of torsion. In other words, if the reflex is absent, it may or may not be torsion. If the reflex is present however, it is unlikely to be torsion.
- Normal cremasteric reflex: lightly stroking the superior medial thigh elicits contraction and elevation of the cremasteric muscle and the ipsilateral scrotum. This is a normal reflex mediated at L1.
- Systemic symptoms favor torsion vs. other diagnosis. This is especially useful when there is diagnostic uncertainty.
- A color-flow Doppler should not delay definitive management and is most helpful in unclear cases such as with long standing, intermittent pain
- Decreased or lack of blood flow to the testicle suggests torsion

Treatment

- The emergency physician may attempt manual detorsion. Turn testis outward and laterally 180 degrees up to 3 times. Classic teaching is to turn the testicle outward like "opening a book." The end point is pain relief indicating reestablished perfusion.
- Definitive management will be surgical exploration, detorsion, and fixation of the tunica to avoid recurrence
- Depending on the source cited, studies indicate that the salvage rate approximates 95-100% when detorsion is performed within 4-6 hours from the onset of symptoms
- Administer opiate analgesics and antiemetics as needed
- The "blue dot sign" in the lateral and superior scrotal wall represents a

cyanotic appendix testis and is pathognomonic for torsion of the appendix testis, a mullerian duct remnant. This is not an emergency and conservative management with analgesics is typically sufficient.

Questions

1. Which of the following favors testicular torsion when there is diagnostic uncertainty?
   A. Dysuria
   B. Gradual pain
   C. Fever
   D. Vomiting
   Answer: D
2. Which physical finding suggests testicular torsion?
   A. The blue dot sign
   B. Lack of the ipsilateral cremasteric reflex
   C. Pain localized to the superior and posterior testis
   D. Pain relieved with elevation of the hemiscrotum
   Answer: B
3. A patient presents with an exquisitely tender and acutely swollen hemiscrotum. You should first
   A. Attempt manual detorsion inward and medially
   B. Attempt manual detorsion outward and laterally
   C. Send the patient for a stat color-flow Doppler
   D. Call urology only if the onset of pain is within 1 hour
   Answer: B

Epididymitis

Critical Knowledge

- An inflammation of the epididymis
- Caused by organisms ascending from the prostatic urethra up the ejaculatory duct, through the vas deferens and into the epididymis
- The typical history is a gradual pain and progressive swelling over several days. Acute onset of pain is less likely and more worrisome for torsion.

- Penile discharge is often present in older and sexually active males
- Systemic symptoms are uncommon and suggest torsion as the leading diagnosis
- Always consider doing a genital exam in patients complaining of abdominal pain regardless of age

Epidemiology/Anatomy

- Etiology is age dependent. In young children, congenital anomalies may result in urinary reflux with a chemical epididymitis or coliform infection. In adolescents and adults age <35, the causative organisms are usually N. gonorrhea and C. trachomatis. Age >35 is usually due to E. coli, pseudomonas, proteus and other coliforms.
- Risk factors include indwelling urinary catheters, recent instrumentation, congenital anomalies of the urinary system, and any activity that increases the risk of acquiring a sexually transmitted disease.
- Pain is initially localized to the posterior and superior poles of the testicle over the area of the epididymis. This inflammatory process may also progress to epididymo-orchitis, resulting in diffuse testicular tenderness thereby making the distinction with torsion more challenging.

Differential Diagnosis

- Same as with testicular torsion

Diagnosis

- Prepubertal epididymitis is rare! Consider congenital anomalies and alternative diagnoses including sexual abuse.
- This is a clinical diagnosis which may be supported by laboratory evidence
- Positive Prehn's Sign: elevation of the involved hemiscrotum alleviates pain suggesting epididymitis. This sign is considered unreliable by itself, and should be used in conjunction with other findings.
- Dysuria, urgency, frequency and pyuria all favor epididymitis vs. testicular torsion
- Increased blood flow on color-flow Doppler suggests epididimytis
- Consider orchitis and inquire about recent infections (post-infectious epididimytis) and immunization status (mumps)

Treatment

- Obtain a urinalysis with culture and a urethral swab for C. trachomatis/ N. gonorrhea cultures
- Treatment for N. gonorrhea and C. trachomatis should be considered as first line treatment for sexually active males and adolescents
- Infants and prepubertal children are less likely to have C. trachomatis/ N. gonorrhea infections and may need to be treated for coliforms as a first line measure. (See UTI section for treatment recommendations).
- Empiric antibiotics for N. gonorrhea include *ceftriaxone* 50 mg/kg/day IV divided q 12 hour. Adolescents can receive the adult dose of *ceftriaxone* 250 mg IM x 1.
- Empiric antibiotics for C. trachomatis include *doxycycline* for children above 8 years of age, dosed at 5 mg/kg/day PO divided BID. Adolescents can receive the adult dose of *doxycycline* 100 mg PO BID x 10 days or *azithromycin* 1 gram PO as a single dose. For children below 8 years of age, give *azithromycin* 10 mg/kg PO x 1 then 5 mg/kg PO x 4 days.
- Consult urology on all young children with epididymitis as there is a high incidence of urinary tract congenital anomalies
- Scrotal support with elevation, NSAIDS, and local ice packs are important adjuncts to treatment
- A common medical pitfall is failure to recognize torsion and failure to treat sexual partners

Questions

1. Which of the following is most consistent with epididymitis when compared to testicular torsion?
   A. Pyuria
   B. Hematuria
   C. Acute onset of pain
   D. Abdominal pain
   Answer: A
2. Young children with recurrent testicular pain attributed to epididymitis should be considered for
   A. Sexual abuse
   B. Congenital anomalies
   C. Intermittent torsion

D. All of the above

Answer: D

3. What is the most common cause of epididymitis in infants and young children:

   A. Gonococci

   B. Pseudomonas

   C. E. Coli

   D. Chlamydia

   Answer: C

Paraphimosis

Critical Knowledge

- A true urologic emergency
- Paraphimosis is the inability to retract the prepuce (foreskin) distally over the glans penis
- Paraphimosis prevents appropriate venous return leading to engorgement of the glans and compromised arterial blood flow. This can lead to ischemia, necrosis and gangrene.
- Causes include infection, masturbation, vigorous sexual activity and urethral foreign bodies. Many cases are iatrogenic during physical examination, urethral instrumentation and with urinary catheters. Hair and clothing tourniquets are important mimics of this diagnosis.
- Complications: penile necrosis with auto-amputation, acute urinary obstruction with risk of renal failure, infection, severe pain
- In contrast, phimosis is the inability to retract the foreskin proximally over the glans. Most cases do not require any form of intervention and simply represent normal human anatomy during infancy. In fact, less than 5% of uncircumcised infants will have a retractable prepuce. This diagnosis is generally a nonemergency.

Epidemiology/Anatomy

- Highest incidence is in infants and adolescents
- Flaccid proximal penis with a collar of swollen and tender prepuce causing distal strangulation, engorgement, pain, and discoloration
- Look for evidence of trauma, irritation, foreign bodies and infection (i.e., cellulitis)

Differential Diagnosis

- Hair tourniquet
- Clothing tourniquet
- Localized urticaria

Diagnosis

- This is a clinical diagnosis based on physical exam findings. Parents will often point out the problem.
- The prepuce will not retract to its normal position over and distal to the glans in the uncircumcised or improperly circumcised male.
- Remember to always examine the genitourinary system as part of the detailed exam of a fussy or crying child, especially when there is no other explanation.

Treatment

- Pain management via topical and/or parenteral route. Options include a topical 2% *lidocaine* gel. Also consider a parenteral analgesic such as *morphine* and a sedative such as *midazolam*.
- Using both of your thumbs, apply gentle and steady pressure on the glans while the other fingers are fixed proximal to the prepuce. Local ice, circumferential manual compression or plastic wraps prior to this procedure help reduce the swelling to facilitate reduction. Success rates are generally very high.
- A dorsal penile block will necessitate a detailed review of a procedure text for the insufficiently experienced hand. One easy approach will involve injecting half *bupivacaine* and half of 1% *lidocaine* without *epinephrine* in either side of the suspensory ligament. A 25 gauge needle is directed into the dorsal base of the penis and towards the anterior and inferior pubic symphysis. Innervation of the penis is by way of the left and right dorsal nerves, both branches of the pudendal nerve.
- For refractory cases, you may attempt an emergency dorsal slit procedure or even the puncture method, although it is recommended that you do these in consultation with urology.
- Consult urology stat from the emergency department for any failed manual reductions or complicated cases. An emergency circumcision may be necessary.
- Do not discharge until you verify that patient is able to void spontaneously.

- Provide teaching on proper prepuce care to parents and patients, along with urology follow up prior to discharge.
- Antibiotics are not routinely indicated unless there is evidence of an infection.

Questions

1. Which is of the following is true?
   A. Phimosis is usually a true medical emergency
   B. Most cases of paraphimosis are successfully reduced without complications
   C. A patient may be discharged immediately after successful reduction
   D. *Lidocaine* with *epinephrine* can be used to perform a dorsal nerve block

   Answer: B

2. Treatment of a paraphimosis may include
   A. The puncture method
   B. Circumferential manual compression of the edematous prepuce while applying steady pressure to the glans
   C. The dorsal slit procedure
   D. All of the above

   Answer: D

Priapism

Critical Knowledge

- This is a prolonged and pathologic penile erection (tumescence) occurring in the absence of sexual stimulation.
- Definitions often describe the erection as lasting over 4 hours, although clinicians should not wait for the 4 hour mark to initiate management.
- There are two types
  1. *Low-flow* (*ischemic*) *priapism* is painful and secondary to decreased venous outflow; this is by far the more common of the two types. It represents a true surgical emergency.
  2. *High-flow* (*non-ischemic*) *priapism* is painless or less painful and secondary to excessive arterial inflow. This is generally not a true surgical emergency although initial expeditious management is still encouraged when there is diagnostic uncertainty.

- Sickle cell accounts for most *ischemic* cases while straddle/groin injuries and spinal cord injuries account for most *non-ischemic* cases. Other causes include leukemia, compressive tumors, illicit drug use, malaria, and medications – especially immunosuppressive agents and intracavernosal injections for erectile dysfunction (usually adults).
- Irreversible tissue injury ensues within 24-48 hours on onset. Without timely management ischemia, necrosis and gangrene occur.
- Remember to always examine the genitourinary system as part of the detailed pediatric exam of a fussy or crying child, especially when there is no other explanation.

Epidemiology/Anatomy

- Distribution is bimodal. The first group is males 5-10 years of age and usually secondary to sickle cell disease. The second group is males 20-50 years of age and most often secondary to medications and drugs.
- With low-flow priapism engorgement of the dorsal corpus cavernosum results in a dorsal penile erection while the ventral surface and glans remain flaccid
- With high-flow priapism there is a semi-rigid shaft with an engorged glans

Differential Diagnosis

- Focus on identifying the precipitant

Diagnosis

- A clinical diagnosis based on a detailed history in conjunction with physical exam findings. Parents and patients will often point out the pathologic erection.
- No imaging studies are necessary to establish the diagnosis, although they help in localizing the problem thereby guiding definitive management. These studies include a color-flow Doppler, MRI, technetium-99m scan, and angiography.
- Consider a complete blood count, reticulocyte count, drug screen

Treatment

- Determine the type of priapism
- Obtain a stat urology consultation
- *Low-flow (ischemic) priapism*: identify and target the underlying disease process

- Administer supplemental oxygen, intravenous fluid hydration, and opiate analgesics as needed
- A dry corpus cavernosum (intracavernous) aspiration may be attempted followed by aspiration with irrigation
- Intracavernous injections with dilute sympathomimetics, such as *phenylephrine*, will exert a potent alpha-mediated arterial constriction
- The use of oral systemic therapies such as *terbutaline* and *pseudoephedrine* are controversial
- Various surgical shunts are used for those who fail initial therapeutic measures
- *High-flow (non-ischemic) priapism:* observation is generally sufficient unless there is diagnostic uncertainty, in which case intracavernous injections and aspiration may be acceptable
- Certain cases may require arterial embolization
- The goal in all cases of priapism is to reestablish normal penile perfusion while preserving function
- Always forewarn parents and patients that complications with or without management include future impotence, although there is a higher incidence with low-flow (ischemic) priapism

Questions

1. Which of the following is not considered a true urologic emergency?
   A. Paraphimosis
   B. Low-flow priapism
   C. Testicular Torsion
   D. Torsion of the appendix testis
   Answer: D
2. Treatment modalities for ischemic or low-flow priapism include:
   A. Dry aspiration of corpus spongiosum
   B. Intracavernous phenylephrine
   C. Intracavernous pseudoephedrine
   D. Arterial embolization
   Answer: B

3. Common causes of ischemic priapism include:
   A. Sickle cell disease
   B. Perineal saddle injuries
   C. Penile trauma
   D. Spinal cord injuries

   Answer: A

References

1. Centers Cherian J, Rao AR, Thwaini A, et al. Medical and surgical management of priapism. *Postgraduate Medical Journal.* February 2006; 82: 89-94.
2. National Guideline Clearinghouse. *Epididymitis. Sexually transmitted diseases guidelines 2006.* Center for Disease Control and Prevention; August 4, 2006.
3. Marx J, Hockberger R, Walls R. Rosen's Emergency Medicine: Concepts and Clinical Practice. The Pediatric Patient: Renal and Genitourinary Tract Disorders; 6th Ed. Philadelphia, PA: Mosby Elsevier; 2006: 2635-2656.
4. Brenner JS, Ojo A. Evaluation of scrotal pain or swelling in children and adolescents. UpToDate website. 2006.
5. Rosenstein D, McAninch JW. Urologic emergencies. *Medical Clinics of North America.* March 2004: 88: 495-518.
6. Wan J, Bloom DA. Genitourinary problems in adolescent males. *Adolescent Medicine.* October 2003: 13: 717-31.
7. Hatzichristou D, Salpiggidis G, Hatzimouratidis K, et al. Management strategy for arterial priapism: therapeutic dilemmas. *The Journal of Urology.* November 2002; 168: 2074-2077.
8. Luzzi GA, O'Brien TS: Acute epididymitis. BJU International. May 2001; 87: 747-55.
9. Blaivas M, Sierzenski P, Lambert M. Emergency evaluation of patients presenting with acute scrotum using bedside ultrasonography. *Academic Emergency Medicine.* January 2001; 8: 90-3.
10. Merlini E, Rotundi F, Seymandi PL, Canning DA. Acute epididymitis and urinary tract anomalies in children. *Scandinavian Journal of Urology and Nephrology.* July 1998; 32: 273-5.
11. Peterson NE. Common urologic emergencies: a logical and practical approach to rapid diagnosis and treatment. *Emergency Medicine Reports.* 1994; 15: 16.

Childhood Asthma (Reactive Airway Disease)

Hans Bradshaw, MD
Departments of Emergency Medicine and Pediatrics
The University of Arizona
Dale P. Woolridge, MD, PhD, FACEP, FAAEM, FAAP
Director Emergency Medicine/Pediatrics Residency Program
Associate Professor of Emergency Medicine and Pediatrics
The University of Arizona

Definition

Asthma is a chronic inflammatory lung disease associated with repeated episodes of airway obstruction and intermittent symptoms of increased airway responsiveness.[1,2]

Diagnosis

Increased work of breathing, cough, expiratory wheeze, hypoxia and clinical signs of respiratory distress. Key clinical signs suggesting a diagnosis of atopy associated with asthma include presence of eczema or dermatitis, seasonal allergies, and a family history of asthma. Differential diagnosis includes: gastroesophageal reflux, rhinitis, aspiration of a foreign body, cystic fibrosis, or structural abnormalities of the upper and lower airways.[2]

Clinical Picture

Initially manifests as reversible airway narrowing resulting in cough, wheezing, dyspnea, and poor air exchange. Increased airway response to various triggering factors such as viral upper respiratory infections, exercise, or environmental stimuli such as cold air, allergens or air pollutants often precede exacerbations.[2]

Pathophysiology

Airway smooth muscle constriction, wall edema, luminal mucus accumulation, submucosal inflammatory cell infiltration, and basement membrane thickening cause airway obstruction symptoms associated with asthma. Bronchoconstriction results in decreased expiratory airflow and is typically reversible with **S**hort **A**cting inhaled **B**eta-2 **A**gonists (**SABA**). Asthma causes **V**entilation-**P**erfusion (**V/Q**) mismatch resulting in hypoxemia. Beta 2-agonists may increase this mismatch due to increased blood flow in areas of the lung that are poorly ventilated. Supplemental oxygen should be utilized to keep saturations of 92% or greater to prevent long-term detrimental developmental effects.[4,5] Chronic inflammation is present in asthmatic lungs making anti-inflammatory therapy such as systemic glucocorticoids essential. Treating or avoiding the underlying triggers for airway hyperresponsiveness can lessen the severity of the exacerbations.

Emergency Department Management

National **A**sthma **E**ducation and **P**revention **P**rogram (**NAEPP**) Guidelines and the American Academy of Allergy, Asthma, and Immunology and the European Academy of Allergology and Clinical Immunology Guidelines.[1,2,3]

Initial Assessment

- ABC's
- Obtain a brief history, past medical history including prior asthma hospitalization course, physical examination (auscultation, accessory muscle use, chest retractions, heart rate, respiratory rate, wheezing, inspiratory to expiratory ratio), **P**eak **E**xpiratory **F**low **R**ate (**PEFR**), oxygen saturation (SaO2), and chest x-ray if indicated to exclude pneumonia or foreign bodies. See Table 1 for normal predicted PEFR values.[6] Consider a white blood cell count, arterial blood gas, and/or electrolytes if severe respiratory distress or altered mental status.

Treatment

- Categorize patients into either: mild-to-moderate (PEFR ≥40% of predicted or personal best), severe asthma exacerbation (PEFR <40%), or impending/actual respiratory arrest.

Impending or Actual Respiratory Arrest Require

- Intubation and mechanical ventilation
- Continuous nebulized SABA (i.e., *albuterol* 0.5 mg/kg/hr if <12 years old and 10-15 mg/hr if 12 years old)
- *Ipratroprium* (0.25 mg every 20 min if <12 years old or 0.5 mg every 30 in if >12 years old)
- Intravenous *corticosteroids* (i.e., *methylprednisolone* 2 mg/kg loading dose then 0.5 mg/kg every 6 hours)
- Adjunct therapies:
  - *Magnesium sulfate* (25-75 mg/kg; maximum dose of 2 g)
  - Antibiotics if comorbid infection such as bacterial pneumonia
- Admit to hospital intensive care
- Electrolyte disturbances (i.e., *potassium, magnesium, and phosphate*) may occur with continuous SABA therapy necessitating serum electrolyte monitoring

- Mild to severe exacerbation patients all get oxygen to achieve $SaO2 \geq 90\%$

Mild-to-Moderate Exacerbation Patients Require

- Inhaled SABA nebulized or by metered dose inhaler (MDI)
    - *Albuterol* nebulized (0.05-0.15 mg/kg <1 year old, 1.25-2.5 mg 1-5 years old, 2.5 mg 5-12 years old, 5 mg >12 years old)
    - MDI with valved chamber (i.e., *albuterol* MDI 90 mcg/act 4-8 puffs) every 20 minutes in the first hour)
- *Oral systemic corticosteroids* (i.e., *prednisolone* or *prednisone* 1-2 mg/kg with maximum dose of 60-80 mg/day)
- If no immediate response to SABA or if recently on oral steroids
    - Repeat assessment including physical exam, PEFR, and SaO2
    - Continue inhaled SABA every 60 minutes for 1-3 hours
    - Make admit decision in <4 hours based on symptoms and PEFR

Severe Exacerbation Patients Require

- High dose inhaled SABA
- *Ipratropium* by nebulizer or MDI with a valved holding chamber every 20 minutes or continuously for 1 hour
- Oral systemic corticosteroids
- If no improvement after intial treatment continue *oxygen*, nebulized SABA plus ipratropium hourly or continuously, intravenous *corticosteroids*, consider adjunct therapies, possible intubation and mechanical ventilation.
- Admit to hospital if incomplete response with PEFR 40-69% predicted/ personal best and continued severe symptoms (i.e., *oxygen* requirement, accessory muscle use, chest retractions)
- Admit to hospital if poor response with PEFR <40% predicted/personal best, partial pressure carbon dioxide (PCO2) ≥ 42 Hg, symptoms including drowsiness and confusion.

Discharge

- Continue inhaled SABA treatment every 4-6 hours for 2-3 days until seen by a primary care physician
- Continue 5-7 day course of oral systemic *corticosteroid*
- Provide patient education (i.e., medication review, inhaler/nebulizer technique training, review/initiate asthma action plan, environmental control measures, insure close medical followup)

- Consider initiation of an inhaled *corticosterioid* (i.e., *budesonide* MDI 200 mcg/act 1 inhalation twice daily if >6 years old with maximum dose 4 inhalations/day, *budesonide* nebulizer for children 1-8 years old with no prior steroid use 0.5 mg/day maximum dose and with prior *steroid* use 1 mg/day maximum dose).

Table 1: Predicted Average Peak Expiratory Flow Rates for Normal Children

Height (cm)	PEFR (LPM)	Height (cm)	PEFR (LPM)
109	147	142	320
112	160	145	334
114	178	147	347
117	187	150	360
119	200	152	373
122	214	155	387
124	227	157	400
127	240	160	413
130	254	163	427
132	267	165	440
135	280	168	454
137	293	170	467
140	307		

Questions

1. Which of the following is not a contributing feature to the pathophysiology of asthma?
   A. Airway smooth muscle constriction
   B. Alveolar spasm
   C. Bronchial wall edema
   D. Bronchial luminal mucus accumulation
   E. Submucosal inflammatory cell infiltration
   Answer: B
2. Medications found beneficial in severe exacerbations of asthma include?
   A. High dose inhaled SABA
   B. Inhaled ipratropium bromide

C. Oral systemic corticosteroids

D. Inhaled corticosteroids

E. Intravenous magnesium sulfate

Answer: D

References

1. National Asthma Education and Prevention Program: Expert panel report III: Guidelines for the diagnosis and management of asthma. Bethesda, MD: National Heart, Lung, and Blood Institute, 2007. (NIH publication no. 08-4051). Full text available online: www.nhlbi.nih.gov/guidelines/asthma/asthgdln.htm (accessed September 1, 2007).
2. Bacharier LB et al. Diagnosis and treatment of asthma in childhood: a PRACTALL consensus report. *Allergy.* 2008; 63[1]: 5-34.
3. Mitka M. New evidence-based guidelines focus on treatment of children with asthma. *JAMA.* 2008 Mar 12; 299(10): 1122-3.
4. Bass, JL, Corwin M, Gozal D, et al. The effect of chronic or intermittent hypoxia on cognition in childhood: a review of the evidence. *Pediatrics* 2004; 114:805.
5. Rodrigo, GJ, Rodriquez Verde, M, Peregalli, V, Rodrigo, C. Effects of short-term 28% and 100% oxygen on PaCO2 and peak expiratory flow rate in acute asthma: a randomized trial. *Chest* 2003; 124:1312.
6. Robertson, J, Shilkofski, N. Harriet Lane: Pulmonology Table 22-3: Predicted Average Peak Expiratory Flow Rates for Normal Children from Voter KZ. *Pediatr Rev* 1996; 17 (2): 53-63.

Bronchiolitis

Hans Bradshaw, MD
Departments of Emergency Medicine and Pediatrics
The University of Arizona
Dale P. Woolridge, MD, PhD, FACEP, FAAEM, FAAP
Director Emergency Medicine/Pediatrics Residency Program
Associate Professor of Emergency Medicine and Pediatrics
The University of Arizona

Definition

Bronchiolitis is a constellation of clinical symptoms and signs including a viral or bacterial **L**ower **R**espiratory **T**ract **I**nfection (**LRTI**) prodrome in children <2 years of age characterized by increased respiratory effort and wheezing not explained by pneumonia or atopy.[1,2]

Diagnosis

Bronchiolitis is diagnosed clinically based upon history of viral upper respiratory illness and physical examination finding of increased respiratory effort and wheezing in children younger than 2 years of age. Typical virologic causes are **RSV** (**R**espiratory **S**yncitial **V**irus), parainfluenza, adenovirus, and influenza viruses. Radiographic or laboratory studies including tests for specific viral agents may support the diagnosis but are not necessary. Radiographs of patients with bronchiolitis typically demonstrate hyperinflation and peribronchial thickening. Per the **A**merican **A**cademy of **P**ediatrics (**AAP**), virologic tests for RSV rarely alter management decisions or outcomes; however, may decreased utilization of antibiotic treatment. An etiologic diagnosis also may be useful if specific antiviral therapy is considered, such as for influenza.[3,4] When an etiologic diagnosis is necessary, the recommended approach is screening by antigen detection or immunofluorescence of respiratory secretions obtained by nasal wash or nasal aspirate (rather than nasopharyngeal swabs)[6]. Rapid antigen tests are available for RSV, parainfluenza, adenovirus, and influenza viruses. Culture and **P**olymerase **C**hain **R**eaction (**PCR**) are additional methods that can be used for viral identification. Differential diagnosis includes: include viral-triggered asthma or wheezing, pneumonia, chronic lung disease, foreign body aspiration, gastroesophageal reflux disease, aspiration, congenital heart disease, heart failure, and vascular rings.[7]

Clinical Presentation

Patients with bronchiolitis often have a 1-3 day history of upper respiratory tract symptoms including rhinorrhea, mild cough, fever, and mild respiratory distress. Physical examination findings include tachypnea (respiratory rate >60–80), retractions (intercostal and subcostal), prolonged expiratory phase wheezing, course lung sounds or crackles, and mild hypoxemia (oxygen saturation Sa02 <95 percent). Patients who are severely affected may have poor feeding, nasal flaring, expiratory grunting, cyanotic appearance, apnea, and poor peripheral perfusion. Other associated findings may include mild conjunctivitis, pharyngitis, otitis media, urinary tract infections.[6]

Pathophysiology

Bronchiolitis is typically caused by a viral infection that affects infants younger than 2 years during the winter. The most common cause is **R**espiratory **S**yncytial **V**irus (**RSV**) followed by parainfluenza virus, human metapneumovirus, influenza virus, parainfluenza, adenovirus, rhinovirus, coronavirus, human bocavirus, and Mycoplasma pneumoniae[8]. Viruses penetrate the epithelial cells in terminal bronchioles resulting in acute inflammation, edema, increased mucus production, bronchospasm, and necrosis of epithelial cells leading to obstruction of small airways and atelectasis. Bronchiolitis is usually self-limited with respiratory status typically improving over 2-5 days.

Emergency Department Management

- Initial assessment: brief history, past medical history including prior respiratory illnesses and course, physical examination (auscultation, accessory muscle use, chest retractions, heart rate, respiratory rate, wheezing, inspiratory to expiratory ratio), **P**eak **E**xpiratory **F**low **R**ate (**PEFR**), oxygen saturation (Sa02), and chest x-ray to look for findings consistent with bronchiolitis and to exclude pneumonia or foreign bodies. Consider a white blood cell count, arterial blood gas, and/or electrolytes if severe respiratory distress or altered mental status.
- Infants whose Sa02 <92 percent should be treated with supplemental oxygen. Antipyretics are indicated if fever (i.e., Tylenol 15 mg/kg every 4-6 hours). Children with tachycardia, copious nasal secretions, dry mucous membranes, and difficulty feeding safely secondary to respiratory distress should be given intravenous fluids. Rehydrate patients with 20 ml/kg bolus of normal saline up to 2-3 times in addition to maintenance intravenous fluids. Nasal suctioning should be preformed on a routine basis if clinically obvious nasal congestion or hypoxic episodes occur. Deep suctioning of the

lower pharynx or larynx is not recommended. Chest physiotherapy is also not recommended unless obvious lobar atelectasis.

- Patients with impending or actual respiratory arrest require intubation and mechanical ventilation with 100% oxygen and continuous nebulized SABA (i.e., *albuterol* 0.5 mg/kg/hr if <12 years old and 10-15 mg/hr if 12 years old). Risk factors for severe disease and/or complications include: gestational age <37 weeks, age <12 weeks, chronic pulmonary disease, congenital heart disease, immunodeficiency, congenital/anatomical defects of the airways, and neurologic disease. Admit to hospital intensive care.
- Patient with mild respiratory distress and hypoxia require a inhaled bronchodilator trial if lower airway obstruction is clinically apparent (i.e., *albuterol* nebulizer 0.05-0.15 mg/kg <1 year old, 1.25-2.5 mg 1-5 years old, 2.5 mg 5-12 years old, 5 mg >12 years old, *epinephrine* 3-4 ml of 1:1,000, or racemic *epinephrine* using a 2.25% solution of 0.05 ml/kg diluted to 3 ml with normal *saline* given over 15 minutes with maximum dose of 0.5 ml/dose). The patient should be reassessed after three treatments spaced 20 minutes apart. Therapy should be discontinued in patients who fail to demonstrate rapid improvement.[9]
- *Corticosteroids* are not recommended in infants with RSV bronchiolitis or pneumonia. In older children, *corticosteroids* may be beneficial in patients with a RSV infection that may have triggered an asthma exacerbation.
- Antiviral *ribavirin* (a nucleoside analog that inhibits RSV) use in infants and children with RSV bronchiolitis is not recommended. *Ribavirin* is expensive and must be given early in the course to be effective. The AAP recommends that decisions regarding the use of *ribavirin* administration should be made on the basis of particular clinical circumstances (i.e., underlying congenital heart disease, lung disease, immunosuppression, need for mechanical ventilation) and clinician experience.[3]
- Antibacterial medications should be used only in children with bronchiolitis who have indications of a coexisting bacterial infection including pneumonia, urinary tract infections, or otitis media.
- *Palivizumab* (a humanized monoclonal antibody against the RSV F *glycoprotein*) may be administered to selected infants and children. The AAP recommends that immunoprophylaxis be considered for certain groups children who are at risk for severe RSV infection. These include infants and young children with BPD, prematurity, and hemodynamically significant congenital heart disease.[1] In addition to these conditions, factors that may influence the decision to administer immunoprophylaxis include the

presence of other conditions that predispose to respiratory illness (e.g., neurologic disease), distance to and availability of hospital care for severe respiratory illness, logistical difficulties of monthly administration and cost. The dose of *palivizumab* is 15 mg/kg intramuscularly once per month for a total of five doses. The first dose is administered before the RSV season begins.

- Prevention of RSV infection includes decreasing exposure to RSV and decreasing the risk of acquisition if exposure occurs. Strategies include: hand decontamination in medical and home settings utilizing alcohol-based rubs or washing, avoid exposure to tobacco smoke, and restricting participation in child care during RSV season for high-risk infants. Families should be educated on the importance of hand sanitation.

Disposition

- The decision for inpatient versus outpatient therapy is based on clinical judgment. Discharging to outpatient followup is appropriate if the child has a good response to rehydration therapy and bronchodilator therapy, tolerates feeding, no oxygen requirement, and no respiratory distress. Discharged patients need to be seen by a primary care physician 1-2 days after discharge.
- Criteria for admission is based on a poor response to rehydration therapy or bronchodilator therapy, a persistently elevated work of breathing, hypoxia (i.e., oxygen requirement secondary to SaO2 <92%), and history of complicating illness such as congenital heart disease, prematurity, or lung disease.[10]

Questions

1. Which of the following is not a risk factor for severe disease in pediatric patients with bronchiolitis?

   A. Acquired disease at ages less than 12 months

   B. History of prematurity

   C. Gestational age at birth of less than 37 weeks

   D. Underlying cardiopulmonary disease

   E. Immunodeficiency

   Answer: A

2. Which of the following is not a treatment option for children with bronchiolitis presenting to the emergency department in respiratory distress?
   A. ABCs
   B. SaO2 monitoring with oxygen therapy to keep >92%
   C. Palivizumab therapy
   D. Rehydration with intravenous fluids if indicated
   E. Trial of inhaled bronchodilators

   Answer: C

References

1. Hanson, IC, Shearer, WT. Bronchiolitis. In: Oski's Pediatrics. Principles and Practice, 4th ed, McMillan, JA, Feigin, RD, DeAngelis, C, Jones, MD (Eds), Lippincott, Williams & Wilkins, Philadelphia 2006. p.1391.
2. McConnochie, KM, Roghmann, KJ. Predicting clinically significant lower respiratory tract illness in childhood following mild bronchiolitis. *Am J Dis Child* 1985; 139:625.
3. Diagnosis and management of bronchiolitis. *Pediatrics* 2006 Oct; 118 (4):1774-93.
4. Bordley, WC, Viswanathan, M, King, VJ, et al. Diagnosis and testing in bronchiolitis: a systematic review. *Arch Pediatr Adolesc Med* 2004; 158:119.
5. Ahluwalia, G, Embree, J, McNicol, P, et al. Comparison of nasopharyngeal aspirate and nasopharyngeal swab specimens for respiratory syncytial virus diagnosis by cell culture, indirect immunofluorescence assay, and enzyme-linked immunosorbent assay. *J Clin Microbiol* 1987; 25:763.
6. Welliver, RC. Bronchiolitis and infectious asthma. In: *Textbook of Pediatric Infectious Diseases*, 5th ed, Feigin, RD, Cherry, JD, Demmler, GJ, Kaplan, SL (Eds), Saunders, Philadelphia, 2004. p. 273.
7. Coffin, SE. Bronchiolitis: in-patient focus. Pediatr Clin North Am 2005; 52:1047.
8. Allander, T, Tammi, MT, Eriksson, M, et al. Cloning of a human parvovirus by molecular screening of respiratory tract samples. *Proc Natl Acad Sci USA* 2005; 102:12891.

9. Langley, JM, Smith, MB, LeBlanc, JC, et al. Racemic epinephrine compared to salbutamol in hospitalized young children with bronchiolitis; a randomized controlled clinical trial. *BMC Pediatr* 2005; 5:7.
10. Lind I, Gill JH, Calabretta N, Polizzoto M. Clinical inquiries. What are hospital admission criteria for infants with bronchiolitis? *J Fam Pract.* 2006 Jan; 55(1):67-9.

English-Spanish Glossary of Common Words

Melissa Zukowski, MD, MPH
Emergency Medicine/Pediatrics Combined Resident
Department of Emergency Medicine and Pediatrics
The University or Arizona

abdomen abdomen (ab-doh-mehn)
abnormal abnormal (ab-nohr-mahl)
abrasion abrasion (ah-brah-see-ohn)
abscess absceso (ahb-sehs-soh)
accident accidente (ag-see-dent-teh)
acetaminophen paracetamol (pah-rah-seh-tay-mohl)
activated charcoal carbón activado (cahr-bohn ahk-tee-vah-doh)
acute agudo (ah-guh-doh)
adolescent adolescente (ah-doh-leh-sehn-teh)
adrenal gland glándula suprarrenales (glahn-duh-lah-suh-prah-reh-nah-lehs)
adult adulto (ah-duhl-toh)
adverse effects efectos adversos (eh-fehk-tohs ahd-vehr-sohs)
age edad (eh-dahd)
airborne en la aire (ehn-lah-aye-reh)
airway vías respiratorias (vee-yahs rehs-pee-rah-toh-ree-ahs)
alcohol alcohol (ahl-coh-hohl)
allergy alergia (ah-lehr-hee-ah)
anaphylactic anafiláctico (ah-nah-fee-lahc-tee-coh)
anemia anemia (ah-neh-mee-yah)
anesthesia anesthesia (ah-nehs-teh-see-yah)
aneurysm aneurisma (ahn-yehr-eehs-mah)
angina angina de pecho (ahn-hee-nah-deh-peh-cho)
antibiotic antibiótico (ahn-tee-bee-oh-tee-coh)
anti-inflammatory antiinflamatorio (ahn-tee-ehn-flah-mah-tohr-ee-oh)
anxiety ansiedad (ahn-see-eh-dad)

appendicitis appendicitis (ah-pehn-dee-see-tees)
arm brazo (brah-soh)
aspiration aspiración (ah-spee-rah-see-ohn)
asthma asma (ahs-mah)
attending physician médico adscrito (meh-dee-coh-ahd-scree-toh)
autoimmune autoinmune (ah-toh-een-muhn)
baby bebé (beh-beh)
back espalda (ehs-pahl-dah)
better mejor (meh-hohr)
biopsy biopsia (bee-ohp-see-yah)
birth nacimiento (nah-see-mee-ehn-toh)
bladder vejiga (veh-hee-gah)
blockage bloqueo (bloh-keh-yoh)
blood sangre (sahn-greh)
blood pressure presión arterial (preh-see-ohn-ahr-teh-ree-ahl)
blood type tipo de sangre (tee-poh-deh-sahn-greh)
body cuerpo (kwehr-poh)
bone hueso (weh-soh)
bowel intestine (een-tehs-teen)
brain cerebro (seh-reh-broh)
breast pecho (peh-choh)
breath, to respirar (rehs-pee-rahr)
bronchitis bronquitis (brohn-kee-tees)
bruise moretón (moh-reh-tohn)
burn quemadura (keh-mah-duhr-rah)
cancer carcinoma (kahr-see-noh-mah)
cardiac cardíaco (kahr-dee-ah-koh)
cellulitis celulitis (sehl-yoo-lee-tees)
cervix cuello uterino (kweh-yoh-ooh-teh-ree-noh)
change cambio (kahm-bee-yoh)
chest pecho (peh-cho)
chicken pox varicela (vah-ree-sehl-lah)
child niño (neen-yoh)

choke asfixia (ahs-feek-see-yah)
cholecystitis colecistitis (cohl-lee-seehs-tee-seehs)
chronic persistente (pehr-seehs-tehn-teh)
clear claro (clah-roh)
clinic consultorio (kohn-sool-tohr-ree-yoh)
cold frío (free-yoh)
coma coma (coh-mah)
concussion conmoción (cohn-moh-see-ohn)
conjunctivitis conjunctivitis (cohn-johnk-tee-vee-teehs)
constipation estreñimiento (ehs-treh-nyee-mee-ehn-toh)
contagious contagioso (kohn-tah-gee-oh-soh)
cough tos (tohs)
CT scan tomografía computada (toh-moh-grah-fee-yah-cohm-puh-tah-dah)
cut incision (een-seh-see-ohn)
death muerte (mwer-teh)
dehydration deshidratación (dehs-hee-drah-tah-see-yohn)
depression depression (deh-preh-see-ohn)
diabetes diabetes (dee-yeh-bee-tees)
diaphragm diafragma (dee-yah-frahg-mah)
diarrhea diarrhea (dee-yah-reh-yah)
differential diferencial (dee-feh-rehn-see-yahl)
digestive tract tracto intestinal (trhak-toh een-tehs-tee-nahl)
discharge flujo (fluh-yoh)
disease enfermedad (ehn-fehr-mee-dahd)
dizzy mareado (mah-ree-ah-doh)
dose dosis (doh-sees)
draw blood, to sacar sangre (sah-kahr sahn-greh)
drug droga (droh-gah)
dry seca (seh-cah)
dysuria distrofia (dees-troh-fee-yah)
ear oído (oh-eeh-doh)
earache dolor de oído (doh-lohr-de-oh-eeh-doh)
EKG electrocardiograma (ee-lehk-troh-kahr-dee-yoh-grah-mah)

elbow codo (coh-doh)
emergency emergencia (ee-mehr-hen-see-yah)
epilepsy epilepsia (eh-pee-lehp-see-yah)
erythema eritema (eh-ree-teh-mah)
eye ojo (oh-hoh)
face cara (cah-rah)
faint desmayo (dehs-mah-yoh)
family familia (fah-meeh-leeh-yah)
feces las heces (lahs-eh-sehs)
female mujer (muh-hehr)
fever fiebre (fee-eh-breh)
finger dedo (deh-doh)
fluid liquido (lee-kweeh-doh)
follow-up recordatorio (reh-kohr-dah-toh-ree-yoh)
food alimento (ah-lee-men-toh)
foot pie (pee-yeh)
fracture fractura (frahc-tuh-rah)
fungal fúngico (foon-gee-koh)
fussy mimado (mee-mah-dah)
gall bladder vesícular biliar (veh-see-kuh-lahr-bee-lee-yar)
gallstone cálculo biliar (kahl-kuh-loh-bee-lee-yahr)
gas flatulencia (flah-tuh-lehn-see-yah)
good bueno (bweh-noh)
green verde (vehr-deh)
hair pelo (peh-loh)
hand mano (mah-noh)
hard duro (duh-roh)
head cabeza (cah-beh-sah)
headache dolor de cabeza (doh-lohr-de-cah-beh-sah)
head injury daño de la cabeza dahn-yoh-de-lah-cah-beh-sah)
heal, to curar (kuh-rahr)
health salud (sah-lood)
healthy sano (sahn-noh)

heart corazón (koh-rah-sohn)
heart attack infarto de miocardio (een-fahr-toh-de-mee-yoh-kar-dee-yoh)
heart rate frecuencia cardíaca (free-kwen-see-yah-kahr-dee-yah-cah)
hello hola (oh-lah)
hematuria hematuria (he-mah-tuh-ree-yah)
hereditary hereditario (heh-reh-dee-tah-ree-yoh)
hernia hernia (hehr-nee-yah)
hip pelvis (pel-vees)
home casa (cah-sah)
hospital hospital (hohs-see-tahl)
hospital admission ingreso en un hospital (een-greh-soh-en-uhn-hohs-pee-tahl)
hot caliente (kah-lee-yen-teh)
hydration hidratación (hee-drah-tah-see-yohn)
hypersensitivity hipersensibilidad (hee-pehr-sehn-see-bee-lee-dahd)
hypertension hypertension (hee-pehr-tehn-see-yohn)
ice hielo (yeh-loh)
ibuprofen *ibuprofeno* (ee-buh-proh-fee-noh)
illness enfermedad (en-fehr-mee-dahd)
immunization vacunación (vah-cuh-nah-see-yohn)
incision incision (ehn-seh-see-yohn)
infant lactante (lahc-tahn-teh)
infection infección (een-fehk-see-yohn)
inflammation inflamación (een-flah-mah-see-yohn)
influenza gripe (gree-peh)
injury lesion (leh-see-yohn)
intensive care cuidados intensivos (kwee-dah-dohs-een-tehn-see-vohs)
internal interno (een-tehr-noh)
intestine intestine (een-tes-tee-noh)
intubation intubación (een-tuh-bah-see-yohn)
irregular aberrante (ah-beh-rahn-teh)
ischemia isquemia (ees-keh-mee-yah)
itch prurito (pruh-reeh-toh)
IV intravenoso (een-trah-veh-non-soh)

jaw mandibula (mahn-dee-buh-lah)
joint articulación (ahr-teek-yoo-lah-see-yohn)
kidney riñón (reen-yohn)
knee rodilla (roh-dee-yah)
lab tests exámenes medicos (ex-ah-mee-nehs-med-dee-cohs)
laceration laceración (lah-seh-rah-see-yohn)
left izquierda (eez-kee-yehr-dah)
leg pierna (pee-yehr-nah)
lesion lesion (leh-see-yohn)
liver hígado (ee-gah-doh)
local anesthesia anesthesia local (ah-nehs-teh-see-yah-loh-cahl)
lung pulmón (puhl-mohn)
lymphadenopathy linfadenopatía (len-fah-deh-noh-pah-tee-yah)
malignant maligno (mah-leeg-noh)
mass masa (mah-sah)
medical medico (med-dee-coh)
medication medicación (meh-dee-kah-see-yohn)
meningitis meningitis (mee-neen-gee-tees)
mild ligero (lee-geh-roh)
moderate moderado (moh-deh-rah-doh)
mouth boca (boh-cah)
muscle músculo (moos-koo-loh)
nausea náuseas (nah-seh-ahs)
neck cuello (kweh-yoh)
needle aguja (ah-guh-hah)
negative negativo (neh-gah-tee-voh)
nerve nervio (nehr-vee-oh)
normal normal (nohr-mahl)
nose nariz (nah-rees)
nurse enfermera (en-fehr-mehr-rah)
ointment pomada (poh-mah-dah)
organ órgano (orh-gah-noh)
outpatient clinic centro ambulatorio (sen-troh-ahm-buh-lah-tah-ree-yoh)